Medicine, Miracles, and Manifestations

A Doctor's Journey Through the Worlds of Divine Intervention, Near-Death Experiences, and Universal Energy

By Dr. John L. Turner

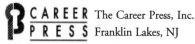

CAREER PRESS   The Career Press, Inc.
Franklin Lakes, NJ

MEDICINE, MIRACLES, AND MANIFESTATIONS
EDITED AND TYPESET BY GINA TALUCCI
Cover design by Ian Shimkoviak, The Book Designers
Printed in the U.S.A.

To order this title, please call toll-free 1-800-CAREER-1 (NJ and Canada: 201-848-0310) to order using VISA or MasterCard, or for further information on books from Career Press.

CAREER
PRESS

The Career Press, Inc., 3 Tice Road, PO Box 687,
Franklin Lakes, NJ 07417
www.careerpress.com
www.newpagebooks.com

Library of Congress Cataloging-in-Publication Data
Turner, John L.
    Medicine, miracles, & manifestations : a doctor's journey through the worlds of divine intervention, near-death experiences, and universal energy / by John L. Turner.
        p. cm.
    Includes index.
    ISBN 978-1-60163-060-5
    1. Turner, John L.—Anecdotes. 2. Neurosurgeons—Hawaii—Anecdotes. I. Title. II. Title: Medicine, miracles, and manifestations.

RD592.9.T875A3 2009
617.4'8092--dc22

                                                                2008053950

To my mother, Dr. Alberta B. Turner,
my father, John Grant Turner,
and President Barack Obama

Acknowledgments

I would like to thank my sister Kay T. Mason who many years ago made me promise to accept a parcel from her with my promise to find 30 uninterrupted minutes to read a *very special book*. In the package was Richard Bach's *Jonathan Livingston Seagull*. That wonderful book allowed me to see how life in this universe may operate. It was the jump-start to my search for an understanding of life, death, and what lies beyond the veil.

I owe thanks to those who struggled through the early drafts of this book. In particular, Mr. Robert Bruce (Australia), author of *Astral Dynamics*, whose groundbreaking work is discussed in the appendix of this book. Thanks to Mr. Martin Simmonds (London), a true friend and brother. I also want to thank Ms. Judy David (Ohio) and Mr. Haywood D. Giles (Ohio), who both made excellent suggestions regarding my early drafts. I feel a special appreciation for a talented artist and friend Mr. Paul Carrick (Boston), who provided the beautiful brain illustrations, and to Professor Linus Chao (Hilo) for the brush and ink calligraphic figures *Heiwa* and *Hikari*. Many thanks go to my good friend Ms. Rosemary Clark (Virginia), author of *The Sacred Tradition in Ancient Egypt*, a brilliant woman who has provided the most excellent guidance. Deep appreciation goes out to Professor Raffi Manasian (California) who helped me see the overall picture, and my friend and agent Jesse Blount, Jr. (California). Thank you, Jesse, for giving me those well-deserved kicks in the seat of my pants to keep me on point.

I would like to thank writing coach and independent editor Mr. Mike Sirota (California), who brought this product to fruition. After all, Sirota is another name for Sartori.

There are not enough words of appreciation to thank Dr. Robert Spetzler of the Barrow Neurologic Institute, Phoenix, Arizona. For a world-famous neurosurgeon of his stature to take time from his busy schedule to read the early form of this book, and to review it again in its final incarnation, was a generous act of "paying it forward." Robert, I thank you a million times for your time and your preparation of the inspirational foreword to the book.

I would also like to thank Dan Jacob. His dandelion animation can be seen on my Website, *www.JohnLTurner.com*. You can see more of Dan's time-lapses on *www.youtube.com* under the user name djacob7.

I thank my wife Mikie Takeuchi Turner and son Doushi for their enthusiastic support.

And last, but certainly not least, I thank Michael Pye and the editors and staff of New Page Books for their assistance and votes of confidence. Because of them, I was able to complete the materialization of *Medicine, Miracles, and Manifestations*.

Contents

Foreword

Neurosurgeons tend to pursue both their vocations and avocations with focus and avidity. To perform surgery on the miraculous and often unforgiving tissue of the brain and spinal cord demands a passionate intensity that inevitably is extended to other pursuits. As readers of this book will discover, John Turner is no exception to this rule. In his case, his outside interest in metaphysics dovetailed with his medical specialty to an exceptional degree and propelled him to explore techniques from complementary and alternative medicine as adjuncts to his rigorous academic and clinical training.

In this articulate and provocative memoir, John recounts his quest to understand the imponderable questions that we all ponder at one time or another—the true meaning of life, whether a spiritual realm exists, the origin of consciousness, and how health and disease might intersect with these aspects of existence. He pursued these questions in the relaxed and welcoming atmosphere of Hilo, Hawaii, becoming the first neurosurgeon on that island. It seems that while Hilo needed him, he, in turn, needed Hilo. There he found the freedom to pursue his individual path to treating patients.

With an open mind and an open heart, John has fearlessly investigated many spiritual disciplines that may be unfamiliar to many readers. Never rejecting his traditional training, he equally fearlessly incorporated whatever healing techniques from these disciplines that he thought might benefit his patients. His success at synthesizing these two approaches readers can judge for themselves.

—Robert F. Spetzler, MD
Phoenix, Arizona
June 2008

Preface

I am a board-certified neurological surgeon, trained at Ohio State University, Columbus, Ohio, and the Cleveland Clinic Foundation, Cleveland, Ohio. My trade involves surgical correction of disorders of the brain, spinal cord, and nerves. The study of metaphysics is among my interests, and it is high on the list of subjects that I plan to master. After 15 years of training in science and medicine, a spiritual path began to unfold as a series of distinct events, some involving patient care and others that were spiritual pathways. With knowledge of metaphysics, one may resolve difficult questions that physical science alone cannot answer. For example, should we believe in powerful gods, as taught by many religious doctrines, or should we realize that a multidimensional energy field creates everything? The facts that support a ubiquitous force are presented as a time-related sequence of episodes that provide corroborating evidence supporting the conclusion that there exists an invisible plane—the spiritual world—where a detailed life plan is created for each of us. The plan outlines lessons we must learn in order to wake to the true situation.

My search began with the desire to understand the meaning of illness, life, death, and life after death. The journey eventually led to alternative methods of treating disease. As I began to understand the mind/body connection, the Hawaiian Islands allowed me to blend Eastern medical techniques of healing with traditional Western allopathic (I use this term to describe "mainstream" medicine) treatments. Hawaii is a melting pot of races and is tolerant of many diverse attitudes and opinions, including the use of complementary and alternative medicine (CAM). In the paradise of Hawaii, I felt free to explore such modalities without opposition or peer pressure.

I took the road less traveled; during the journey, I explored many pathways leading to perfection of the spirit. All of them were informative and enlightening. I will present these pathways to you as a series of experiences that appeared to follow a script.

It was inevitable that alternative methods of healing would present themselves along the way, because such techniques involve the mind, body, and spirit. For a physician and surgeon, such additional tools offer the best possible chance to overcome disease. However, equally important in treating illness, if not more so, is treating the patient.

Introduction

When I began my medical practice in Hawaii, my preparatory training consisted of a degree in engineering physics, a medical diploma, and several years of postgraduate training in neurological surgery (the study of the nervous system and how to repair it). For me, armed with expertise in physics and neuroscience, everything was in place to understand the mind/body connection. Medicine and metaphysics are continuing themes that play a role in each chapter of this book; as far as miracles go, the miraculous events began the day I set foot on the island of Hawaii.

At the start of my awakening, I received the call to action from an astonishing report generated from a computerized version of the ancient *I Ching*, the *Book of Changes* developed in the century before Confucius. While sitting at my computer in 1995, I thought of asking a question. I wanted to know if things were going in the best possible manner and if I was following the right path in life. Many mysterious events had occurred throughout the past several years and I felt as if something extraordinary was about to take place—a significant change of some sort. The prophetic result can be summarized as follows:

Question: *Am I on the right track?*

Response: *Enormous potential*

"Great power becomes even greater when it is harnessed and held in check. Like a river that has been dammed, the restraint of power produces enormous potential. If one's actions are benevolent and are in alignment with the 'general good,' one's creativity will be rewarded with immense success. In political or business affairs, it is a time to assert leadership. But be forewarned: success can turn to failure if strength turns to arrogance."

After pondering the meaning of this report, I decided it was time to commence writing this book. The early chapters explain what guided me into metaphysics. I wondered why I had been chosen to work with the human brain, to understand its intricacies, and to repair it when injured. Was it fate or was it by choice? Born into comfortable circumstances, I had the freedom to set out on a search for why, how, and where: why we are here, how it came about, and where we go after our last breath is taken. My investigation involved medicine, miracles, and manifestations. When I realized that near death experiences (NDE) and out of body experiences (OBE) were fact and not fiction, I became resolute in continuing to investigate the true meaning of existence. The heart of my search was to answer several key questions: are we brief candles, strutting and fretting on the stage of life, only to be extinguished when the play ends? Do we live time after time in a continuously expanding and never-ending universe? Do we have free will or are we preprogrammed and guided every step of the way? And finally, how do we remain healthy and whole so that the experience may be completed and enjoyed?

This is a factual story of transformation—changes that taught me how to rise above preconceived notions and prejudices to see the great beyond. It is about spiritual enlightenment, innovative methods of treating disease, and a path to perfect understanding.

After completing the six-year neurosurgical training program at the Cleveland Clinic Foundation in 1981, I wanted to embark on my surgical career far from the chaos of Cleveland, Ohio. The multicultural and multiracial aspect of the Hawaiian Islands suggested that Hilo, Hawaii would be an idyllic place for me to live. I didn't know at the time that in the Hawaiian language, Hilo means "to twist." Indeed, personal strife—including the second and third marital divorces—gave me more than just a twist. In Japanese, Hilo can be translated as, "A swirling vortex of fire." From the physical aspect, the Kilauea volcano—a scant 35 miles from Hilo—has been erupting constantly since January 1983. My personal travels were, metaphorically speaking, constantly twisting in various directions and accompanied by much heat and fire. From the metaphysical standpoint, I found that I had to twist my way through the fire to become spiritually clean.

During the tough years of medical school and neurosurgical training, I gained a new family, and my wife and our two young sons accompanied me on the flight to Hilo. Looking out the window, seeing the endless stretch of billowing clouds, I recalled my first trip to Hawaii just three months before. On that occasion, I came to interview for the position as neurosurgeon with the Hilo Medical Group. I sat with a young married couple who loved Hawaii. They told me stories of their yearly trips to the islands and how great it had been for them.

"That's your island," the man said as we began our descent into the Honolulu airport. Out the window in the far distance, 200 miles beyond Oahu, I could see two large gray humps of land poking through the cloud layer. These were the huge volcanic mountains of *Mauna Kea* and *Mauna Loa,* which formed the Big Island of Hawaii. During the flight, I told my seatmates that the Big Island had, until now, been without a neurosurgeon. I would be the first to service the island in this regard—should I decide to take the job. My companions remarked about my good fortune and said that they were genuinely happy for me.

I'll always remember that first visit to Hawaii—stepping off the plane, I found myself immediately falling in love with the island and its people. The Big Island reminded me of the years I spent in Puerto Rico as a petty officer in the U.S. Navy; fields of sugar cane and swaying palm trees now surrounded me once again. The deep blue color of the ocean and the light blue sky generated familiar feelings of peace and serenity.

When I arrived at the airport on that first occasion, a light rain greeted me. A Hawaiian rainbow, my first, arched over the airport parking lot. Dr. Adler, a pediatrician at the medical group, was assigned to pick me up. This smiling *haole* (I didn't know this Hawaiian word for a white person at the time) drove me to my hotel, The Naniloa Surf. The medical group had spared no expense in providing a room with an ocean view. I opened the drapes to see the vast expanse of the Pacific Ocean with mountains in the background arching skyward to more than 14,000 feet. What a gorgeous day! I turned on the radio, hoping to pair this splendid visual scene with fitting musical accompaniment, and I was not disappointed. As if on cue, I heard the song *Mahalo e Hilo Hanakahi.* I had no idea what that meant, but I later learned that it translates roughly as, "We give great thanks to you, Hilo." I also learned the story told by the Hawaiian words. The song speaks of the warmth and friendliness of the people of Hilo, the beauty of the forests and flowers, and that newcomers are always welcome. I immediately put my suit and dress shirts, along with two ties, directly into the wastebasket. I knew instinctively that Hilo would be the place for me.

Now, on my second trip to Hawaii with my family, I gazed at the Big Island from the port windows of the Boeing 747, and my eyes welled with tears. It was as if I were returning to a lover after a three-month separation.

We arrived in time for the local Independence Day celebration. The downtown area in Hawaii's second-largest city was alive with merriment. I felt at home, relieved to be wearing flip-flop sandals, shorts, and colorful Aloha shirts. Hilo was a place where the races mingled in a melting pot that radiated harmony and peace. I felt out of harm's way here, and sensed that in this place of majestic beauty, I could achieve new levels of self-knowledge and a connection with nature.

My spiritual path began in graduate school when I read Edgar Cayce's story *The Sleeping Prophet,* by Jess Stearn, one of many books that would significantly affect the course of my life. Mr. Cayce, a man of average intelligence and little formal education, enjoyed a particular gift: he could place himself in a trance state and extract information about illness, alternative medical treatments, and many other subjects from an unseen dimension in time and space. This was a fascinating book, so engaging that it soon led me directly into the office of the curriculum adviser of the physics department to change my major from engineering and physics to medicine. I became captivated with the thought of a spiritual world and I desperately wanted to find it.

I had to put my search for the unseen spiritual dimensions on hold as it was time for me to think about employment as a neurosurgeon, now that my training was complete. I recalled how I'd traveled from New York to California in search of a position where living conditions would be conducive to the normal growth and development of my two young mixed-race sons, sparing them from ethnic turmoil. But after I had given up hope of finding a suitable place to settle, I picked up the *Journal of Neurosurgery* one April morning in 1981, just two months before my training would be complete. Inside, I found an article with bold headlines:

Neurosurgeon wanted—Hilo, Hawaii.

Excellent opportunities for sailing, skiing, and surfing.

Contact The Hilo Medical Group.

Hilo, Hawaii.

"Sailing, skiing, and surfing" were not what attracted me. *Wanted* was the first of two keywords that caught my attention, as it had a sense of urgency to it; the second was *Hilo*. Was coming to Hilo an episode in my life that had been written, as if I were following a script? Whatever the reason, Hawaii provided a comfortable environment for my family. My children and I looked like locals; we felt a sense of belonging. As a man with a multi-racial background (German, Irish, American Indian, and African blood), I had not been exposed to racial mixtures in my hometown of Columbus, Ohio. There, you were either black or white; there were no in-betweens. The Midwest had not been kind. Hilo was the place for me. I was married to a Caucasian woman, and interracial marriage was commonplace in Hawaii; nobody seemed to care.

During the two years following my beginning the practice of neurosurgery (starting my first night on call with a case that encouraged me to study the spiritual world), I found little time to spare for anything but the demands of my profession. What little time that remained I devoted to the study of metaphysics. Having frequently witnessed death and dying, my interests remained focused on the meanings of life…and of death.

Two illustrative surgical cases presented themselves in close proximity. The first was that of Mrs. Ibarra. This experience suggested that there is a force that we can summon on command when we need assistance. However, the second case, Sara, made me wonder if there was any such force at all.

Chapter 1

Divine Intervention— God Giveth, God Taketh Away: Mrs. Ibarra's Gift

Hold off your hands...and know that I am God.
—Psalm 46:10

I n operating room 3, the only audible sounds were the soft
wheeze of the anesthesiologist's respirator and the occasional
soft click of instruments being passed between rubber-gloved
hands. Through the lenses of the operating microscope, I could
clearly see the magnified stereoscopic images of Mrs. Ibarra's brain
tumor, a large peach-sized outgrowth of the *dura* (a thin leather-
like membrane) that covers the brain. This benign lesion was
behind this 72-year-old woman's right eye; total removal would
be a cure. For the past four hours I had been slowly, but steadily,
removing the growth piecemeal—the hard way—with electric
forceps and wire-cutting loops (small circular heated wires on
the end of a plastic wand). As the loop sliced through the tumor,
smoke and vapor obscured the field. My assistant, Dr. Peterson,

sucked the smoke away with his metal suction tip. I longed for the ultrasonic aspirator that I had used in training; it would have made this job much easier.

Four hours had elapsed since Mrs. Ibarra's surgery began and I had one remaining portion of tumor left—a small, scraggly clump of cells at the bottom of the operative field, hardly bigger than a pencil eraser.

"Just one little piece remaining," I told Dr. Peterson. He could see it too; he had an excellent view through his observer's eye-pieces. I easily sliced through the remaining tumor with the cutting loops and then suddenly, like an explosion, the field of view turned bright red.

"Suction!" The nurse complied, placing the tool in my hand.

Eventually, through the process of suctioning away the obscuring blood, I came to a startling realization: the last small piece of tumor had invaded the *carotid* artery, the major artery supplying the right side of the brain. The overlying tumor cells hid this fact from me. Removal of that final portion had taken out a section of the artery's wall; without applying pressure to seal it off, the vessel would bleed profusely. I initiated repair of the vessel.

"Silver clip," I commanded. The nurse handed me long-handled clip-applying forceps.

Because of the invasion by the tumor, the clips would not take a solid grasp; no matter how many times I tried, they didn't work.

Dr. Flower, the anesthesiologist, said, "Are you going to get it? I've given her three units of blood."

"The carotid artery has cut loose; I have to repair the arterial wall," I replied. Dr. Flower returned to his position at the head of the table behind the drapes. "Suture, eight zero," I requested as I continued to peer into the microscope lenses. I began the slow and tedious process of sewing the vessel, but was confronted with another problem: the walls of the artery were softened by the tumor, and the suture would not take a solid grip but merely pull through when tightened, causing further injury to the vessel.

I repeated my efforts with clips and sutures while minutes multiplied. I had spent four hours trying to stop the blood loss. Dr. Flower replaced the woman's entire blood volume with donor blood; she was now a candidate for developing dreaded complications that can result after massive blood transfusion. My patient had been under general anesthesia for more than eight hours and had received 10 pints of blood. I was nowhere close to being finished. It appeared as through I were about to experience my first loss of a patient during surgery, and would be introduced to the feeling of having caused a patient's death. I should have foreseen the possibility that the last remaining piece of tumor was a sticky wicket and just left it alone.

All eyes in the operating room were on me. All ears waited. What was I to do? I had exhausted all of my options...all but one! I never thought of praying before this day. Although I had been an acolyte in the Episcopal Church as a youth, I had no interest in religion. Having trained in physics, I doubted the significance of prayer and was skeptical about the existence of God. I had been too busy with academics during the past 21 years to allow time for religion. But today I prayed with sincerity. I would have fallen to my knees if I had not been scrubbed in and sterile.

I felt incapable of saving the life of this patient. I took a deep breath and exhaled slowly. I needed to connect with that force. As I looked through the scope, I prayed silently: *If there is a God, a higher power, then I need your help. It is not Mrs. Ibarra's fault that she may die. I have done all that I can do. I am asking for help. Don't let her die on the table; help me to repair this damaged artery. Please!*

I took a second deep breath…and went back into the breech.

"Suture," I said. For what seemed to be the umpteenth time, the scrub nurse obeyed my request. Once more, I carefully tried to approximate the torn vessel's walls.

"Clip," I said. She handed me clip after clip until, after 15 minutes, I had applied several clips and snippets of suture, trying to bring the remaining walls of the artery together without occluding the vessel. To my amazement, the operative field remained as dry as a bone! No bleeding. I was pleasantly stunned. I'd done nothing out of the ordinary during that last 15 minutes except to repeat the previous attempts of the past few hours. But this time, the sutures and clips held firm. The prayer—the silent plea—had worked. The damaged artery showed no sign of bleeding. Everything at the base of the skull looked perfect.

"We're out of here," I told the scrub nurse and my assistant. All that remained was to close the operative site. This took 45 minutes, but it was a walk in the park compared to the ordeal I had faced over the past nine hours. Now, believing that my prayers had produced the miracle, I put forth another silent request: *I have one more favor to ask. Please do not let her be comatose. Let her wake up and heal quickly. Do not let her become stroked out and paralyzed, but instead let her speech and strength be normal.*

Let her come out of this in the best possible way. If you do this, I'll be as good a person as I can possibly be.

When helping to move her from the operating table for the trip to the Intensive Care Unit, Dr. Flower said, "You know, you have to learn that you can't make 'good enough' better."

This case taught me that there is a higher power. It had seemed to flow through me when called upon. Was this the God who created us in His image? Alternatively, was it a force, an energy that is available when summoned to supercharge our meager human efforts? At the time, I was unsure just what to call it. It was there waiting for my call, and when asked, it came to my assistance. Although signs pointed to God, a nagging question bothered me. Was it something within *me* that required the slow, deep breathing and mental refocusing for its activation? Whatever the mechanism, it was now a moot point—Mrs. Ibarra was going to at least make it to the ICU and I would be forever thankful. Now if she could just pull through intact, I would be the second-happiest person on the island.

Mrs. Ibarra not only survived the surgery, but she healed quickly with little neurological sequelae. She was discharged in seemingly normal condition one week later. Besides *ptosis* (a slight droop) of her right eyelid, she had a second problem. I found out about it three months after surgery when she came to my office for a final post-operative checkup.

"How is your eye?" I asked.

"Oh about the same, doc," she replied, "I've learned to live with it, and it's not bad at all. But I have a problem. My husband will not give me enough sex!" She smiled at me, and I smiled back. That was a great complaint for a woman in her seventh decade of life.

"I don't think I can help you with that," I replied. "Are there any other physical problems?"

"Not really. Say, I have something for you, doctor." She pulled a large piece of lacquered wood from her shopping bag. On it were two engraved Japanese *kanji*. The patient, however, was from the Philippines. I was confused. The Japanese characters must be of special importance.

"What is this?" I asked. "What does it say?"

"Oh, I don't really know, I'm not Japanese. But when I found it, I had the feeling that somehow, in some way, doctor, it was for you. This is what you need."

"Well, thank you very much. I will treasure it and think of you often."

She smiled again, and I returned her smile in kind.

"This is your last visit with me, Mrs. Ibarra. You have done well; the scan we did last week reveals no further tumor growth; in fact, the scan was normal. I will recommend to your doctor that he perform a follow-up scan in six months to confirm that everything is still okay. If you have a question or would like to see me, please call anytime."

Later on, I asked a few of my surgical colleagues if they had experienced a case where they could not stop the bleeding. The response was uniformly, "Yes, why?"

"What did you do?"

And again, the reply was always the same: "What *can* you do?"

At the end of the year, I hosted a Christmas party at my office. During the festivities, I pulled my friend Dr. Nagashima aside and showed him the calligraphy that Mrs. Ibarra had given me. "What does that mean?" I asked.

He peered at it for a moment through his thick eyeglasses. "Heiwa," he said. "Roughly translated, it means peace."

And indeed, as a result of my intraoperative prayer, Mrs. Ibarra survived. Now that I knew a higher power was with me, I was at peace, confident that I could overcome any difficulties either on my own or with help, on those rare occasions when good enough truly needs to be made better.

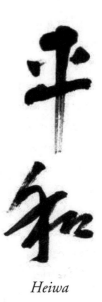

Heiwa

Sara's Sudden Demise

Every life has dark tracts and long stretches of somber tint, and no representation is true to fact which dips its pencil only in light, and flings no shadows on the canvas.

—Alexander MacLaren

I continued to bask in the blissful feeling of serenity that resulted from the prayerful experience that ostensibly saved the life of Mrs. Ibarra. I augmented my budding conviction in the unseen spiritual world (and a higher power) when I became "born again" at a local Pentecostal church. I'd connected with the universal force (that I now called God), and felt as if I could ask it to aid me at any time. I became filled with the Holy Spirit. Time passed, until an otherwise routine day changed dramatically into one of the saddest days of my life. It was an experience that caused me to rethink my recent religious conversion and to search for another answer to the mysteries of life and death.

Sara DeAngelo came with her parents for a consultation. Nine years old, she radiated great beauty and spirit. Her smile was adorable and by her appearance and manner, I could tell that one day she could potentially be a fashion model. She had been blessed with great looks. I was struck by her natural charm and her soft-spoken, friendly nature, seemingly years beyond her age. Her parents worked in the sugar industry and had recently moved to Hawaii. The girl had a ventriculoperitoneal shunt—a bypass tube with a valve that drains cerebrospinal fluid (CSF) from the brain to the abdomen to treat hydrocephalus (enlargement of the fluid spaces of the brain). The shunt was performed in the first days of her life. There had been no problems with the device since its insertion, but in time, she would outgrow the length of tubing in her abdomen and it would have to be replaced. Shunts also can become obstructed.

Shunts come in many varieties. The most common type is a flexible silicone catheter that is inserted into the brain. This is done by placing a small hole in the back of the head and inserting the catheter into the ventricular fluid system deep within the brain. A valve mechanism allows one-way flow of CSF from brain to abdomen. Tunneled under the skin, a discharge tube allows drainage into the abdominal cavity. Babies born with "water on the brain" suffer from CSF buildup when egress from the ventricular cavities of the brain is blocked. A pressure-relieving procedure must be performed quickly. Sara had such a shunting procedure after birth and had done well.

Sara conversed with me easily and submitted to a neurological examination without duress. Her parents were pleased as they observed our interaction, and at the end of the consultation they requested that I be available should the shunt require surgical treatment. I agreed and told them how to contact me in case of emergency. I scheduled an X-ray to estimate the remaining length of tubing. As a result, I determined that she could grow a few more inches in height before modification would be necessary. I admired this little girl and mused about someday having a child of my own as sweet as Sara DeAngelo.

Everything stayed quiet for many months. Then one day, the emergency room called. Sara had suddenly become seriously ill with complaints of severe headache and came to the emergency department for treatment. A CAT scan showed obstructive hydrocephalus with her ventricular system under high pressure. The shunt was blocked. I arrived at the hospital within minutes to find the mother holding her retching child over a sink in the X-ray department, suffering from the increased pressure in her head that, if untreated, would soon lead to brain herniation as pressure forced brain tissue through the opening at the base of the skull. Coma and death would quickly follow. My evaluation showed the shunt to be occluded at the valve; I planned to insert a new system. I explained the procedure and its risks to the parents and they requested that surgery be done. Within the hour, I was scrubbing for surgery.

In the operating room I glanced at the monitor; her respiratory and heart rates were normal. The anesthesiologist waited for me to begin. I put on gown and gloves and went to the table.

"Knife," I said. The nurse gave me the necessary scalpel and I opened the old incision, disconnected the valve and—suddenly, without warning, the ventricular catheter fractured and disappeared into the brain.

"Damn it!" I exclaimed, perhaps a little too loud.

It had been old and brittle. To retrieve it could cause injury to the brain and might stir up bleeding that could be difficult or impossible to control. It was better to let it float forever within the ventricular chamber. I inserted a new system without difficulty and made sure that it properly drained the fluid drop by drop. I closed both incisions and applied sterile dressings. Sara went to recovery and then to the pediatrics unit, her room directly across from the nursing station. The nurses would keep a close eye on her. Sara's father planned to spend the night in her room. I told him of the difficulty with the old tubing breaking off and disappearing within the brain, and of my decision not to try and recover it. He understood.

I returned home that evening feeling good about the surgery. Before retiring, I called the pediatric floor. Sara was reported to be sleeping comfortably with normal vital signs.

"Remember to check on her routinely as ordered."

"Of course doctor," the nurse replied, "she's doing just fine."

I awoke with a start at 6 a.m., rubbed my eyes, and wondered about Sara. I had slept through the night without a phone call, so apparently she was doing well. Showering, I mentally reviewed my schedule for the day: office appointments were the only tasks after morning rounds. I would have preferred surgery, as office evaluations tend to be tedious, although necessary, drudgeries.

Suddenly, the phone rang. It was my answering service. "Code Blue Pediatrics, doctor, your patient!"

I could not believe it. I threw on a scrub suit and ran to my car. I lived only a mile or two from the hospital and I arrived within minutes to face a flurry of activity in Sara's room. The on-call anesthesiologist was there with several nurses and a crash cart of medical supplies. The child was intubated; a machine ventilated her lungs.

I grabbed a hypodermic needle from the cart and inserted it quickly through the scalp and into the shunt valve. Maybe the new shunt had malfunctioned or the old ventricular catheter had caused an obstruction and buildup of fluid pressure. To my amazement, there was no sign of high pressure. Only a few small drops of fluid came from the needle. The valve has a plastic portion that can be pumped with using thumb pressure—it operated normally. I lifted her eyelids; her pupils were fully dilated and did not respond to light. This was an ominous sign of brain death. Sara was transferred to the intensive care unit. I spoke with her dad, who had just walked into the room.

"What happened?" he cried.

"I'm not sure. Can you tell me how it went during the night? The nurses report that she had a peaceful sleep until just before six this morning when they found her comatose and unresponsive."

"I spent the entire night with her," he said slowly, crushed by the rapidity of recent events and the now critical condition of his daughter. "She whimpered occasionally and complained of mild pain where you made the incisions, but all in all, I was quite pleased with her progress. I thought it would be okay to run down for a cup of coffee. When I returned, the room was filled with doctors and nurses. They said her heart stopped."

As we walked to the ICU, I told Sara's distraught father that I wanted to do a brain scan to see if the shunt was decompressing the ventricles and if the old tube had somehow caused damage, bleeding, or obstruction. He consented, and we went from the ICU to the CT scan with Sara. The scan was normal. Sara remained comatose with fixed and dilated pupils. She had no history of cardiac or any disease other than the aforementioned hydrocephalus at birth.

I sat by the bedside holding her hand, thinking and rethinking this case. Would I have done anything differently? Should I have sent her to the ICU after surgery with a special monitor in case her breathing stopped? No, the pediatric nurses were always on top of things, and her room was directly across from their station. There was really no need for special monitoring. Should I have tried to recover the lost tubing from the ventricle? No, that may have caused more problems.

"Doctor, may I begin?" said Thomas Bearden, the brain-wave technician, as he prepared to wheel his electroencephalograph (EEG) into the room. This test would confirm brain death.

"Of course," I said. As he attached the scalp electrodes using conductive paste, I turned to look out the window. The parking lot was slowly filling up as doctors arrived to begin their daily ritual of morning rounds. It was quiet in the room except for the occasional hiss of the ventilator as it kept Sara's lungs and blood well oxygenated.

After Thomas finished, I saw that the recording was flat line (no electrical activity) at the highest sensitivity setting of the machine. There could be no question about brain death, an irreversible condition in spite of the continued beating of her heart and mechanical inflation of her lungs.

I gave the parents the sad news. I told them I had no idea how or why their daughter died suddenly. I requested an autopsy. Maybe it would reveal if the catheter was the cause of her death. In addition, it might have disclosed an unknown heart condition that could have led to cardiac arrest. I needed to know the etiology of her demise.

"Doctor," the father said, "we understand your concern *and* your pain. It may be that we will never know what happened. Although an autopsy may help you to understand, we have carefully thought this out. We would prefer, as would Sara, that she be an organ donor. Her heart, liver, kidneys, and eyes may give someone else a better life. My wife and I sincerely believe this would be her wish."

"Are you sure? There is a chance the old tubing may have—"

"Please doctor," he interrupted. "I really do understand your concern, and we empathize with you, but we feel the most benefit will be to donate her organs."

I wiped a tear away. It was indeed a sad day to see this beautiful child gone from the world. Yesterday, she had been her normal cheerful self, dressing for school, when she began to complain of a headache. By the afternoon she had started to vomit, a result of the pressure developing within her brain. Now it was over. I was dumbfounded and unable to understand this fatal series of events.

The organ harvest team took Sara to the operating room. Her heart, lungs, liver, and kidneys were deemed suitable for donation, as were the corneas of her eyes. As she was wheeled from the room, I sighed in grief, lowered my head and gave Sara a silent farewell.

A few days later, the parents called to invite me to a funeral event for Sara, which they called a "Celebration of Life." As I drove the 50 miles to the small church, I again pondered the case. If I had to do it over I would do the same thing: leave the old tube, nurse the patient on the pediatrics floor, and leave the same routine orders for post-op nursing assessment. I would feel comfortable, even if it were my child. Would this ever happen a second time? It could, as medicine is an art as well as a practice. But I sincerely hoped that I would not have to face such a tragic situation again. I arrived at the church in time for the celebration of life.

"We thank all of our family and friends for coming today," the mother said. About 50 or more friends and relatives had gathered for the event. "We want to say how fortunate we feel to have had Sara in our lives for the past nine years. She was truly a gift from God and provided us with untold joy and happiness." Her remarks were followed by a message from the father and brief remarks from a few friends of the family. The service ended with a meal of local-style food and drink. I offered my condolences to the family and left.

The universal force, the higher power that came through with Mrs. Ibarra, was unaccountably absent in Sara's case. I was more than disappointed. I felt deeply saddened and baffled. I decided to continue my investigation of a spiritual world to determine if there was such a thing as a universal force. It is of note that years later, when I observe my 3-year-old son laughing and playing, and when seeing how he fondly looks at me, I can't help but wonder, *could this be Sara?*

Chapter 2

Welcome to Paradise

Well, I've often felt that dreams are answers to questions we haven't yet figured out how to ask.

—Fox Mulder, *The X Files*

I suggested there was a God that could be called upon at a time of need. But the case of little Sara DeAngelo—although I'd felt no need for assistance—seemed to indicate that this God would, at times, turn his or her back and become seemingly indifferent to human suffering. How could this be? It is said that God is *just*. Now I could not help but wonder, *just* what is God?

My Hawaiian introduction to the spiritual world began two years before my encounters with Mrs. Ibarra and Sara. The wheels in that heavenly dimension began to turn with full force the first night I was on call in Hilo, and the circumstance surrounding this baptismal immersion is something that I will never forget. Due to a tugboat and shipping strike, my ordered surgical equipment had not arrived. Not having the requisite tools for brain surgery was going to put a serious crimp in my practice, but I convinced myself that the ships would soon sail and the equipment would arrive. To my dismay, destiny had no plans to deliver my instruments any time soon. Instead, with the cards stacked against me, putting me against all odds, fate sent Jordan Kalapana calling.

"Doctor," said a pleasant voice from the answering service, "I have the emergency room on the line."

My pulse began to quicken. A moment later, I heard the voice of the emergency room doctor: "Hello Jack. This is Dr. Bodine. We're going to need your help."

"Absolutely," I responded. "What's the problem?"

"I have a young man who was riding his dirt bike in the forest and was thrown off, striking a utility pole's guy-wire headfirst. Unfortunately, he was not wearing a helmet. I've checked him over, and his right pupil is dilated. We've done skull films and there's no sign of a fracture."

"All right," I said, "I'll be there in a minute. Type and crossmatch him for two units of packed red cells."

The dilated pupil indicated that his brain was being forced out of the bottom of the skull, compressing the third cranial nerve and dilating the pupil. The next thing to happen would be compression of his brainstem and that would be "all she wrote."

I drove lickety-split to the hospital. In the ER, the central desk was empty, not a doctor or nurse in sight at the computer screens. An eerie quiet blanketed the scene; the only sounds were those of soft footsteps as two nurses scurried between curtain-obscured rooms. I stopped one of them.

"Excuse me," I said, "where is the head-injury patient?"

"Are you a relative?" she asked. "I'm sorry but you will have to wait. I'm busy now."

"Nurse," I said a bit testily, "I'm a neurosurgeon."

"Oh…I'm sorry doctor." Her manner suddenly changed to one of respect. Being Japanese, she bowed politely and added, "Your patient is in room 6; I'll get his chart for you and alert Dr. Bodine that you're here." She handed me the chart from the nursing station. "We are so happy that you're here, doctor. We've been praying for a neurosurgeon. I'll be right back." Bowing one more time, she disappeared down the hall.

Not knowing what to expect, I entered ER room 6, parted the curtains with my hands, and stopped short—the familiar conditions I had learned to expect after years of training were missing. *Was I in my right mind to take this job?*

The injured teenager was semi-comatose on the gurney, a stack of blood-soaked gauze pads taped onto his head. He took an occasional gasping breath and his right hand pulled at his shirt as if he had an itch.

"Do you have cervical (neck) films?" I asked the nurse.

"No doctor, we only have skull films." She flicked a switch and the view box came to life, showing a lateral view of the head with an obvious linear fracture of the skull.

Adrenaline is a funny thing. A surge of it will get you moving, like it or not. I felt the surge. "Get an intubation tray quickly," I said. "And call for a stat lateral neck film."

"Certainly, doctor." She left through the curtains, nearly bumping into another nurse who had just entered.

"Where is Dr. Bodine?" I asked?

"He just woke up, doctor. He should be here in a second," she replied, wringing her hands anxiously.

"His head is stabilized, doctor," an orderly said after he finished placing sandbags alongside the patient's head, and securing them with adhesive tape.

"I can put in the bladder catheter for you, doctor," the nurse offered. I nodded; she began the catheterization.

"Dr. Turner?" The emergency room physician could barely stifle a yawn. I removed my gloves and shook his hand. He was an older man, a temporary hire from Nevada. He wore a white coat that was rumpled and stained. He rubbed his eyes and then beamed at me broadly.

"You'll never know how glad we are to have you here," he said, echoing the first nurse's sentiments. "I know nothing about how to treat this. In the past, our only option was to fly such patients out to the nearest neurosurgeon in Honolulu. This, of course, resulted in a critical loss of time, sometimes several hours. You are a godsend Dr. Turner, and we thank our lucky stars you've joined us."

With all the praise being lavished on me, I decided not to chastise him for neglecting to perform basic resuscitation and triage procedures. Hilo's doctors and nurses had never been forced to deal with neurosurgical trauma. If they could ship the patient out, they would do so as quickly as possible. If the patient died before transfer, there was little that they could have done to prevent it.

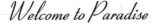

The wall phone rang; it was the operating room nurse. I told her, "This is Dr. Turner. I have an emergency. It will be a craniotomy…right parietal, for subdural hematoma."

"I'll find what I can for you, sir, but we have only a few of the instruments listed on your card."

"Get together as much as you can and tell me how much longer until I can bring him up to surgery." I glanced at the clock. "He's about to die," I added quietly.

"I am sorry doctor, but we don't have a night staff in-house. The girls are on call at home. Some of them live 30 minutes away."

"Okay," I said, recognizing the futility of getting angry. "Then move as fast as you can."

After checking all the lab work and quickly writing up the examination results, I spoke with the patient's mother, who had been brought to the hospital. The boy had been identified as Jordan Kalapana, age 19. His mother was anxious to speak with me. After calming her down, I explained that time did not allow us to fly him to Honolulu for a CT scan and surgery. His brain was herniating due to pressure, and there was no time for angiography (an X-ray study of blood flowing through the brain). I would have to operate immediately, basing my approach on the high probability that the blood clot was on the same side as the dilated pupil and the skull fracture.

"Will he live, doctor?" she asked me, anxiety flooding over her gentle face.

"Mrs. Kalapana, I'm afraid the situation is critical, and if your son is to have any chance at all, I must proceed quickly with decompression. The odds are against his making it. I would say that at best he has one chance in ten to survive the operation."

"Please do what has to be done, Dr. Turner." She wiped away tears from her eyes. "I trust you." Her remark surprised me. During my years of training, no patient or family had ever remarked that they *trusted* me. I made a mental note to look into this further when time permitted.

"I will do my best, Mrs. Kalapana," I told the Hawaiian woman, meaning every word.

A nurse appeared. "We're ready for you doctor." I directed Mrs. Kalapana to the waiting area and told her that I would keep her informed by relaying messages through a nurse.

At 10:30 p.m. I donned a green scrub suit for the first time in Hawaii. I again wondered what neurosurgical equipment, if any, would be available. I gamely put on a mask and entered the operating suite.

The patient lay belly up on the operating table with an anesthesiologist seated behind his head, adjusting his equipment. When he saw me enter the room, he stood to shake my hand.

"I'm Dr. Turner," I said, "and you are…?"

"Why, hello there," the smiling physician responded. "I'm Joe Bob Pelt. I'll be doin' the anesthesia for y'all." Dr. Pelt, a mainland transplant, talked as if he had taken a belt of sour mash whiskey from a Mason jar. I would soon discover that he was a highly skilled anesthesiologist in spite of his country demeanor.

A dozen assorted surgical instruments were laid out for my use—mostly hemostats and needle holders. After positioning the patient, I picked up and examined a hand drill that looked like a

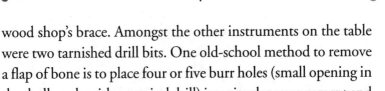

wood shop's brace. Amongst the other instruments on the table were two tarnished drill bits. One old-school method to remove a flap of bone is to place four or five burr holes (small opening in the skull made with a surgical drill) in a circular arrangement and connect them using a wire saw (a Gigli). The faster way is to use a power drill and power saw.

"Can you get the Gigli saw handles and blades?" I asked the nurse.

"Gigli what?" she asked, looking at me like I had just spoken to her in Swahili.

"You know, the tool I need to cut through the bone." I made sawing motions with my hands.

"I'm afraid we don't have anything like that, Dr. Turner," she said. "We have never had a case like this before."

"Well, do you have any other bone removal instruments?" I tried not to sound irritated.

"No, doctor, only this one," she answered, pointing to a small rongeur, a pliers-like instrument used for removing small portions of bone.

"This is going to be rough," I mumbled. I could probably remove enough bone with the hand drill and rongeur to get out the clot, but it would be a slow process.

I looked at young Jordan. He was near death with a traumatic clot on his brain. I glanced at the small tray of hemostats and needle holders; my gaze followed the nurses as they rushed about looking for various items and suddenly, it hit me full force: *I was in the boondocks!* I took a deep breath and thought, *this was what you wanted, and this is what you got.*

With great effort, I drilled through the bone of the skull. Taking the rongeur, I chipped away at the skull, removing small bits of bone until I had removed a section measuring 2 inches in diameter. The dura was now exposed. The dark purple color and drum-like tightness indicated that thick-clotted blood would be found underneath. I cut open the dura and removed a large collection of jelly-like clot. The effect of the blood, which had compressed the brain without the buffering protection of the dura, was causing his brain to well up with pressure. Joe Bob gave him medications; eventually the swelling subsided and I was able to close the dura, suture the scalp, and end the case.

"We're very appreciative," the scrub nurse told me afterward. "You did your best with crude equipment. The shipping strike will end soon and you'll have your modern instruments."

"Thank you. I hope he will survive, but it doesn't look good for him."

I spent the next few days closely watching the boy. I had no electronic intracranial monitor to measure the pressure within the skull. I could estimate intracranial pressure by feeling the tension on the scalp over the bone opening. It remained firm. On the second day, a small amount of brain tissue oozed from the wound margins. Both of the boy's pupils dilated fully and became fixed to light (no reaction). He showed no ability to breathe on his own. He became respirator-dependent and brain dead.

Although there was no EEG equipment available at the time to confirm the diagnosis, I surmised him to be clinically dead based on examination and the fact that he could not initiate breathing. My recommendation to the family was to discontinue life support, as I saw no chance for recovery. However, the family could not agree on a decision to disconnect the respirator. Many were in favor of doing so, but some wanted to wait a few more days. I could only advise; the family had to decide.

The night of the fourth post-operative day, I experienced a strange dream in which I was making rounds in the ICU and came to Jordan's bedside. As I watched his face, he suddenly triggered the machine and started breathing on his own. I awoke with a start. The clock read 4 a.m. I called the ICU, but the nurse reported no significant change in the boy's condition; he remained unresponsive and ventilator dependent. In fact, his blood pressure had shown wide intermittent fluctuations on both sides of normal. His temperature had increased in spite of cooling blankets and medication. He was not improving; he was going further downhill.

When making rounds that morning, I stopped by Jordan's bed and spent time watching him. His eyes were closed, and tears flowed slowly down his cheeks, most likely byproducts of the autonomic nervous system, rather than tears of sadness or pain. Still, one never knows for sure.

"Doctor, he took one breath just before you arrived," his nurse said, interrupting my thoughts.

"What was that?" I asked sharply.

"We saw him trigger the respirator, but it was brief. We called your answering service, but you were on your way here. Just before you came in he took another breath on his own."

"Amazing." I told her of my dream. "Keep a close eye on him and reduce the machine to 10 breaths per minute." I thought

I could let a little carbon dioxide build up to stimulate his breathing, but alas, my dream was not to be realized. During the next two days, Jordan showed no further signs of respiratory effort. His blood pressure became increasingly unstable. I performed an apnea (suspension of breathing) test that showed that he was unable to take a breath after temporary disconnection from the respirator. This was disheartening. The dream had been so vivid and encouraging, and shortly after my dream, Jordan had taken a breath or two. I felt sad that his recovery was not to be.

In view of the results of the apnea test, the family asked me to discontinue life support. They bade him farewell, each in their own way. I turned off the machine; in less than 30 minutes, his heart stopped beating and he passed.

A few days later, I received a call from Jordan's father, who had just arrived from California. He asked to see me to discuss his son's death. He stressed the fact that he wished to speak with me in person, "face to face," and "eye to eye."

I told him to come by at 4 o'clock. He agreed, and at the appointed time a handsome Hawaiian man appeared at my door. I was more than happy to discuss the details of his son's demise with him. "Mr. Kalapana," I began, "we did everything possible for your son, but under the circumstances, the extent of the head injury was such that there was little we could do...little that *I* could do as a surgeon." We were now face to face.

"I understand that my son visited you?"

"No, I'm afraid not. The first time I saw Jordan was the night of his injury."

"I'm talking about your dream," he said. I looked at him, shocked.

"How did you know about that?" I asked, amazed that he knew about my dream experience.

"One of the nurses told me."

"Mr. Kalapana, I wish I could tell you the dream was prophetic. The next day your son took a few breaths, but unfortunately, he was unable to continue breathing on his own. I'm sorry."

"That's not the point." He leaned toward me, until we were indeed eye to eye. "Let me tell you why I came to speak with you in person. No one questions your ability or the fact that you did all that was possible for my boy. We Hawaiians have strong spiritual beliefs. We did not interpret your dream as a sign that he would recover."

"How, then?" I asked, puzzled.

"To us it is a sign that he contacted you. His spirit made contact so you would understand that he did not want his life prolonged with machines. He wanted to be free to continue his journey. He wanted you to let him go."

I sat back, my mind trying to grasp the meaning behind his words. The father patiently waited for me to speak.

"That's certainly possible," I admitted. "I may have misinterpreted the dream. I took it as a sign of recovery…but now that you mention it, the dream may have prompted me to perform the breathing test and again approach the family about stopping the ventilator. Still—"

"Exactly," Jordan's father interrupted. "That is what we believe. I thought it would be important for you to understand this concept, as it will play a major part in your work." He stood, shook my hand and added, "There are those who make things happen; those who watch things happen; and those who don't know what the hell happened. You are destined to make things happen for Hilo." He thanked me for helping his son, then turned and walked out the door.

I thought deeply about my meeting with Jordan's father. The man traveled from California to speak with me in person, as if what he had to say was too important to trust to the phone; his message was about the spirit world and Hawaiian beliefs. I had completely missed the meaning of the dream. The true significance had not been obvious; the visit from Jordan's father gave me a different perspective. Was the dream evidence of a spiritual world, as the man had implied? And had Jordan somehow contacted me so I could allow him to move beyond death?

I had no answers. At that moment, I decided to study the true meaning of death. I began with Dr. Raymond Moody's work on near-death experiences (NDE). There must be an answer, and I became determined to search for it; this seemed to be an appropriate starting point. I had little trouble finding books on NDE; the library and bookstores were replete with texts on astral projection (something familiar to me from college days) and near-death experiences.

As I studied these materials, it became clear that many patients who nearly died often reported a series of distinct stages. The first was being out of their bodies and floating up to a corner of the room, then observing with detached interest as doctors and nurses conducted the resuscitation. They could often recall the equipment used, medications given, and conversations overheard. This was followed by a trip through the "tunnel" and into the "light" where they were greeted by previously departed

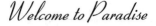

loved ones. There was often a life assessment: a complete three-dimensional pictorial review of the past life's events. They were given the option to continue with the process or to return to the body. It was comforting to know that the experiencers had not wanted to come back, as the journey was blissful, but because of family or other obligations, they reluctantly returned to their bodies. Conceivably, the unsuccessful resuscitations involved a willful choice to continue on death's path.

As I studied NDE reports carefully, I began to realize that we have a spirit that does not extinguish at death, but lives on to begin a new journey: we are more than just a physical body. Jordan's dream contact suggested that this was correct. Was there any way that things could have worked out differently for him, or was this his fate? The next case shows that perhaps—just perhaps—one's destiny *can* be changed.

Chapter 3

The Mysterious Case of Mrs. Dahm Luk

Today is the tomorrow you were worried about yesterday.
Was it worth it?

—Siddhartha

Jordan Kalapana's passing jump-started my search for the meaning of illness, life, and death. I read as much as I could about the astral plane and near-death experiences. I wondered if illness could be defeated by a conscious effort to alter the mind/body connection. Was there a way to manipulate health on the astral plane? Little did I know that an extraordinary example of this would appear as the next piece of the puzzle and that as a bonus, the messenger would be an African-American Zen monk named John Hall.

It was late September, several weeks after my meeting with Mr. Kalapana. The previous day had been a rough one for me, in the operating room and emergency room most of the time, and it took only a moment to fall into a peaceful slumber. After what seemed like minutes, the nonstop ring of the phone woke me up.

"Dr. Turner," the ER doctor said, "I have a 58-year-old man who suffered a brief loss of consciousness after an auto accident. He has a one-inch scalp wound, and he's alert and oriented. However, I'm concerned about the loss of consciousness. Would you mind taking a quick look at him?"

"I'm on my way," I replied.

Hilo Hospital did not have a CT scanner; I was the next best choice. What I thought would be a routine consultation turned out to be an integral part of my spiritual education. After arriving at the hospital, I faced a mysterious stranger in the ER. The patient sat on a gurney, a small gauze pad taped to his head. He smiled warmly when I entered the room. I introduced myself as the neurosurgeon called for consultation.

"Hello, my brother," he said. I realized from his smile, his firm handshake, and the way his eyes locked on to mine, that we would be friends. The teaching is that strangers are merely family that one has not yet met. I had this feeling with John.

The ambulance report stated that he admitted to losing consciousness; his first memory after the impact was the ambulance attendant prodding him for his name. He felt fine now, except for pain on the left side of his clean-shaven pate where the bandage covered a small cut. I examined him neurologically, finding no evidence of brain or nerve injury.

"I think you'll be just fine. I'll give you a head sheet (home-care instructions given to head-injured patients), which will tell you what to watch for throughout the next 24 hours. In your case, the risk of brain bleeding is small. Before you go, I want to place a few sutures through that cut."

"That's not necessary, brother," he said, "I'll leave now. Thank you for your kindness."

"You can't go yet, I need to sew you up."

"Is it still bleeding?"

"No, the bleeding has stopped."

"Then I can leave."

"Hold on a minute." I restrained him with my hand. "I think sutures will close the scalp edges nicely and in time, the injury will be barely noticeable."

"Let me explain why I prefer to allow it to heal as it is," he said. "You see, I must have created bad *karma*. Now I must pay the price. If it heals leaving a scar, then I must accept this as my karmic payback—my karmic retribution."

"You did something that resulted in your injury?" I asked.

"Indeed," he replied. I wanted to question him further, but I decided to wait.

He stood, smiled, and extended his hand. "Thank you, doctor. I'll remember you."

"How will you get back to your car?" I asked.

"I can walk."

"Walk? Why, that's about 4 miles."

"This is my karma," John said.

"Listen John, I insist that you let me drop you off." I told him that my wanting to help must also be part of his karma. He agreed, unable to argue with that logic.

On the way to his car, we talked. John had come to Hawaii from Nashville and married a Japanese woman many years younger. They had two small boys. He beamed radiantly as he passed a family snapshot to me. The children of mixed race were beautiful. They reminded me of my sons who were nearly the same ages. John, a singer and musician, recounted several years spent in a Zen monastery, striving to become enlightened. He came to Hilo to begin a new life.

We made plans to meet again, and in time, through John's music, I became interested in keyboards and other instruments. More importantly, John always spoke of "doing good deeds" and having only "good thoughts." They called him Brother John, or sometimes "Buddha John," because of his bald head and his proselytizing on Hilo streets. He gave impromptu lectures in local coffee shops, stressing the importance of right thought, right action, and right intention.

I didn't have to wait long for the next significant meeting with Brother John Hall. It happened two years later.

That auspicious day, I pulled into the parking lot, exited the car, and rushed to the elevator. I was 30 minutes late for work; hospital rounds had held me up. As the only neurological specialist, I found it difficult to make rounds and leave the hospital without having to do an urgent consultation.

I entered my office and faced a waiting room full of patients. Nodding in acknowledgment, I apologized for making them wait, and then went into the back office, where the pleasant smile of Brother John greeted me from the couch where he sat.

"Hello friend," he said. We embraced warmly.

"Aloha John, it has been a long time. How have you been?"

"I've been great," he replied with a grin. Suddenly, his expression changed to one of deep concern. "My friend, Mrs. Dahm Luk, is not so great. She's here to see you for consultation and I've accompanied her…with these." He pulled a set of CT scans from the X-ray envelope in his lap and handed me the films. Holding them up to the light, I saw a large midline tumor within the *corpus callosum*, the bridge of connecting fibers between the hemispheres of her brain.

"She's waiting in your exam room," John said.

"All right John, let's talk to her. This is a cancerous tumor." John nodded that he understood.

Mrs. Dahm Luk, a middle-aged Vietnamese woman, was fidgeting with the buttons on her blouse when we entered the room, her eyes darting to mine and then back to her feet. Her anxiety was understandable. I was sure that she sensed this was a point of transition; she was about to face a serious problem.

Her two daughters sat with her and after John introduced me, I took her history and performed a physical exam. She suffered from headaches for the past two months and because of persistent complaints, her family doctor ordered a brain scan. I put the films on the view box. I told them the lesion—about the size of a lemon—was a malignant growth because of its central location, appearance on the scan, and the rapid increase in her compliants of headache. Removal was out of the question, as it involved the crossing fibers connecting the halves of her brain. Any attempt to remove or debulk this lesion would drastically affect her neurologic condition by causing a disconnection syndrome. Strange and disabling neurologic symptoms would result. The proper treatment would involve a biopsy followed by radiation therapy for several weeks. After that, she would need chemotherapy to give her any chance of survival. I was unable to paint a hopeful picture.

"The biopsy will involve performing a craniotomy to expose the brain and then working between the hemispheres to obtain a small piece of the tumor. After we confirm the diagnosis of cancer, radiation and chemotherapy may help to extend your life."

She looked apprehensively around the room and then discussed the situation with her daughters. They agreed with my treatment plan and encouraged their mother's consent. Mrs. Dahm Luk gave in to my recommendations. I called my assistant Leilani into the room and told her the details of the surgery I intended to perform. She took notes, then left to make the necessary arrangements.

"Well that's about it," I said, bringing the meeting to a close.

"Thank you, doctor," said the patient. John gave me a thumbs-up sign and said he would talk to me after the operation.

The delicate surgery went well and there were no complications. A piece of tumor went to pathology, and, as expected, the tumor was malignant (an astrocytoma). It was not the highest grade (astrocytomas are graded I to IV, the higher the number, the more the aggressive tumor), but it was headed that way. It didn't look good for her. After a few days to heal from the surgery, she would begin the first of seven weeks of radiation treatments. I told the patient and family of the dismal prognosis and that at best, treatment might extend her life for a few months to a year. Her postoperative course was uneventful, and she left the hospital with instructions to come to my office the following week for suture removal.

On the appointed day, Mrs. Dahm Luk arrived at my office with her daughters, John, and seven Vietnamese Buddhist monks wearing bright yellow ceremonial garb. They made an attractive group. Leilani had removed the sutures and the incision looked good. I reviewed the brain scan taken after surgery. There was no sign of bleeding or any new problems. The tumor continued to stand out like a light bulb in the center of her brain. I wanted to see her again after radiation therapy. A repeat scan would show the result of treatment. I told them I hoped to see a decrease in the size of the tumor. This was as positive as I could be. Mrs. Dahm Luk was a woman with one foot on a banana peel and the other foot in the grave; that banana (her last connection to life on Earth) was slowly sliding from beneath her foot.

After they left, John requested we step into my office for a chat. "I'll bet you think those monks traveled from Vietnam to pray and chant for her, don't you, brother?" he said. I nodded and said it appeared that way to me. "Well, I want to tell you that you're wrong."

"John, come on. They have the *juzu* (prayer) beads and they wear the saffron-colored costume; it's my bet that they came to pray for her."

"No," John said. "I want to tell you what is happening. For the past seven days, they have taken her through a guided meditation. During that experience she saw her soul in one of the seven hell worlds, where she suffered torments as a hungry ghost for seven days while suffering in flames." He rubbed the side of his head, remembering his injury, and then continued. "The cause of her suffering was obvious. She harbored hatred for a lady friend and held this inside for many years. Because of its intensity and ferocity, this hate manifested as illness; the result was her brain tumor. The monks work with her day and night to allow her to recognize the karmic significance of her hatred and to persuade her to forgive. She must release her evil thoughts connected with this woman. If she can let go of the hate, she can heal—the tumor will leave. Her mind and body will then be at ease rather than *dis*-ease."

"John," I said, "I have yet to see a malignant brain tumor cured by radiation, chemotherapy, or surgery. The word itself means "disposed to do evil." Many patients with this problem resort to prayer to help them. However, try as they may, a malignant tumor is fatal."

"Friend," he continued, "it's not prayer, but karmic understanding that the monks are providing. Her negative feelings have set into motion a cause-and-effect process that has taken its toll on her body; the tumor is the result. If she can understand the karmic connection, if she can forgive and *truly* forgive, she can heal. Sure, the radiation can help, but without her giving up the hate she harbors, it will have no effect."

I thought about what he said as I continued to watch the man. In his late 50s, he was a slender fellow in great physical shape. A strict vegetarian and family oriented, he conducted a Buddhist service monthly for members of a small congregation not far from town. He'd spoken of karma during our first meeting, and again he was speaking about it. I looked at his head: the wound was barely noticeable. Something made me want to believe him, but my Western medical training held me back.

"I have doubts about it, John. I wish her the best, but I'm afraid she doesn't have long to live."

After John left, I looked out the window at Hilo Bay. Gentle waves lapped at the breakwater in the distance on this sunny morning. Maybe it was karma that brought me to Hawaii and karma that brought me to John. I would soon have the answers, and I would witness one method by which spontaneous healing may occur.

I realized that karma was a credible reality five weeks later when the entourage of patient, family, and monks appeared in my office for a follow-up visit. Radiation therapy was over and Mrs. Dahm Luk looked like a healthy 63-year-old woman.

"Let's have a look," I said, removing the latest scan from the package. As I placed the films on the viewer, I mentally debated which oncologist I might engage for chemotherapy. I flicked the power switch that provided backlighting.

"Whoa!" I was sure there was a mistake. Did these scans belong to another patient? There was no tumor on the films. I couldn't believe my eyes! There was no trace of the lesion that had glared menacingly from the screen before and after surgery. I examined the date, name, and hospital number on the films. Unmistakably, these scans were Mrs. Dahm Luk's, taken yesterday, *and there was no tumor.* In fact, other than the surgical evidence of my drilling and cutting bone, the scan looked normal. It was incredible!

I called the radiologist who read the films and asked for his opinion. He said that he had to do a double take and then a triple take because of the surprising absence of the tumor. He was present during the scan and when the films came from the processor. No mistake in marking the films: they belonged to

Mrs. Dahm Luk. I asked him if he had seen anything like this before and he said that he had not.

"Well," I told the group, "I'm happy to report the radiologist and I concur—the tumor is gone. If there are residual tumor cells, they are too small to detect by CT scanning. For now, consider yourself cured."

They smiled and nodded at one another, but there were no whoops of joy. It was as if they had known the result all along. They thanked me, and before leaving, scheduled a follow-up visit and repeat scan in six months. John also thanked me, but he did something else: in his quiet way, he smiled and winked at me as if saying, *See how it works?*

After they left, I sat reviewing the scan in quiet contemplation. Seven monks, seven weeks of radiation, and seven Hell Worlds? In Christian theology, triple sevens are throught to represent perfection and holiness. There seemed to be a seven connection in Buddhist philosophy as well. Here was a case of emotional disarray that when corrected, allowed healing to take place. Was it the patient's realization or belief in the karmic cause of her disease that allowed her brain to join with radiation to expel the foreign invader? According to John, she released all negative feelings about the other woman. Were surgery and radiation necessary at all? I paced back and forth in my office, pondering the matter. There may be countless individuals who have experienced similar lesions that never came to the attention of a doctor, and healed because of faith. Could most human illness be psychosomatic? Astral plane, near-death experiences, and karmic retribution—there must be some principle at work, some pathway that I can uncover, to connect the dots and explain how such medical miracles take place.

I heard that the patient lived several more years in Hilo and then died after returning to Vietnam. I didn't know if her death was because of a recurrent tumor or another cause. I cannot remember her first name, but I like to think of her as Mrs. Bess Dahm Luk. The reason? Because either she was an example of the workings of the spiritual world, or she had the *best damn luck* that I had ever seen! Either way, call it luck or karmic resolution, it was a first for me. It altered my thinking about disease.

Chapter 4

Soul Travel

I am not discouraged, because every wrong attempt discarded is another step forward.

—Thomas Edison

The spiritual experience with Mrs. Ibarra, the disastrous death of Sara DeAngelo and the surprising healing of Mrs. Dahm Luk acted as catalysts to speed up my study of illness and the spiritual world. Mrs. Dahm Luk's cure demonstrated that working with karma on the astral plane was a powerful tool with which we could fight disease. My next step was to explore those otherworldly dimensions.

During my years at Ohio State University, I loved reading about astral projection, but I was unsuccessful escaping from my body. I now turned my attention to Sylvan Muldoon and Hereward Carrington's *The Projection of the Astral Body*. This is a classic on the astral plane, and a must read for anyone interested in the subject. For NDE, another must read is *Life After Life*, by ɹr. Raymond A. Moody. When Dr. Moody was a medical student, a patient who recounted a near-death experience came to his attention. He was fascinated by the patient's description of the NDE. Word of Dr. Moody's interest spread quickly and led to more referrals, and eventually, his first book on out-of-the-body experiences.

NDE travelers described the first stage of the journey as a realization that they were out of the physical body watching the resuscitation efforts. Many recalled specific words used by the doctors and nurses present, the names of drugs and the equipment used, and more. A series of events followed, including a past-life review where everything that had occurred in the person's life was shown to them visually, as if watching his or her entire life in a three-dimensional presentation. There were more steps in the process and some, but not all, described travel through a dark tunnel and into the light. In the light, they were greeted by their ancestors and previously departed loved ones. A common element in the reported experiences was that they were given chances to continue the journey or return to their physical bodies. In fact, because of the blissful feelings they experienced, most wanted to continue on, but because of obligations on Earth (family and loved ones), they reluctantly agreed to return. After having a pleasurable near-death experience, any fear of death they held before was gone.

Although the majority of near-death experiencers had pleasant and often rapturous travels, a small percentage had "hell-like" encounters with demons and monsters. There may be many more we don't hear about that were horrific; after all, who would like reporting that they went to hell?

I gathered as much written information as I could about resuscitation-related NDEs, but considered it imprudent to seek such patients. I was pleasantly surprised when two of my patients voluntarily spoke to me about it, describing the near-death experiences in detail. How and why did these experiences occur, and more importantly, what was behind going into the light? It raises an interesting question: When the occipital lobe (visual center) of the brain is deprived of oxygen and glucose, could the resultant nutrient deficiency cause the light-related experiences? Many scientists offer this as the explanation.

Is there a portion of the brain that generates near-death events as chemically induced hallucinations at the time of death or serious illness? Yes, there are electrochemical explanations. When portions of the temporal lobe are stimulated electrically or magnetically, subjective experiences involving light are generated. Those with a religious background may see visions of Jesus, Buddha, or Mohammed, correlating with their particular beliefs. Conversely, those with a strong interest in extraterrestrials may see the bright white light of a spacecraft.

In a September 2002 article in *New Scientist,* Swiss researchers (University Hospitals of Geneva and Lausanne) reported that stimulation of the right angular *gyrus* of the brain (in the parietal lobe) produced the "floating out of the body" sensation. It is conjectured that this area of the brain is sensitive to drops in blood pressure (something that could occur during anesthesia and surgery) and could generate NDEs.

In his book *DMT: The Spirit Molecule—A Doctor's Revolutionary Research Into the Biology of Near-Death and Mystical Experiences,* Dr. Rick Strassman hypothesizes that DMT (dimethyltryptamine), a short-acting but potent psychedelic, may be produced by the *pineal* gland. The pineal is situated in close proximity to the superior and inferior *colliculi* of the brain, a place where important auditory and visual connections are made. The release of this chemical into the CSF (which bathes the collicular plate) could also explain the white light sensations.

In the prestigious *New England Journal of Medicine*, Dr. Dirk De Ridder, department of neurosurgery at the University Hospital Antwerp, in Belgium, was able to reproduce OBE by stimulation of implanted electrodes near the temporoparietal junction (a region necessary for reasoning about *the beliefs of others*). The electrodes had been implanted in their patient for intractable tinnitus (ringing of the ears). The doctors were experimenting with a new type of signal generator and were surprised by the 17 seconds of OBE, which could be produced on a repeatable basis when the electrodes were energized. Using positron emission tomography (PET) scans, they were able to pinpoint activation of the angular-supramarginal gyrus junction and another area, the superior temporal *gyrus-sulcus*, on the right side of their 63-year-old patient's brain.

My attempts to personally experience an out-of-body state were unsuccessful. Although the books I read offered hints, suggestions, and techniques about how to do it, I could not separate my mind from my physical body. I realized there was more to life, death, and spirit that I needed to understand. As if according to plan, the next episode was not only just around the corner, it was next door. What you are about to read describes either a mysterious science, or the fabrications of a highly imaginative mind: the writings of Paul Twitchell.

Not long after I began my study of the spiritual world, I went to collect the day's mail and as I returned to the house my neighbor, Dr. Bob Klein, spotted me and invited me to chat. Surprisingly, one of the first things he said was, "Have you heard of Eckankar? It is called the ancient science of soul travel."

"Soul travel? No I haven't, Bob—why do you ask?"

He pointed to the letters in my hand: on top of the pile was a newsletter from A.R.E., the Association for Research and Enlightenment, devoted to the study of Edgar Cayce's readings. I was a card-carrying member and Bob had noticed the mailing envelope.

"I see that you have an interest in the paranormal," he said. "I have studied Eckankar for years. Come in for a second; I have a book that might interest you." We walked into his house, where he handed me a book and said, "I think this is what you are seeking."

He was right about that. I was looking for a doorway to the spiritual world that would open and allow me to enter. The book he gave me was *Dialogues With the Master* by Paul Twitchell. The cover depicted a man seated at a desk, paper before him and pen in hand. A dark-skinned, bearded man stood next to him. Dr. Klein told me that Mr. Twitchell was receiving dictation from one of the "ECK Masters," the Tibetan, Rebazar Tarzs.

I thanked him for the book and promised to contact him after I finished reading it. I thought it exceedingly strange to be holding a book that told a tale about the nightly ethereal appearance of Rebazar Tarzs in Twitchell's bedroom. The information transmitted during sessions with Tarzs dealt with the tenets of

Eckankar, a strange religion. Eckankar was brought to public attention in 1965 by Mr. Twitchell who, under the tutelage of the prior ECK Masters, trained to become an ECK Master.

I read the writings of Twitchell with interest. Either this was true or it was a great entertaining work of fiction. It was similar to the trance-state readings of Edgar Cayce—messages from another plane and another dimension. Eckankar teaches that humans are on a spiritual sojourn, a path seeking God realization based on the eternal existence of the soul. Contact with the Divine Spirit (ECK) and astral soul traveling with a "teacher" to places of higher learning were the mechanisms whereby one could explore the spiritual world. I was interested in the Eckist's tripartite concept of "The Spirit, the Sound, and the Light of God." Bob Klein had been correct: this was *exactly* what I had been looking for—a means by which I could investigate the spiritual world. My goal of metaphysical training appeared close to realization.

I visited the Eckankar bookstore in Honolulu and purchased several books. According to Twitchell, the astral plane consists of 150 regions. There are upper levels accessible from the Earth plane by means of "soul travel," a means to reach the higher Causal and Mental levels. To me, soul travel was identical with astral projection. I ordered a series of 12 monthly exercises, each one describing a different method of "rolling out of the body" to enter the OBE state. I began to chant the sacred word of the ECK planes and quietly vocalized the Eckist's sacred name for God, which is *Hu*. I decided to give Eckankar one year of study.

Along with the writings of Twitchell, I read Robert Monroe's *Journeys out of the Body*, and coupled his teaching with those of Eckankar in hopes of promoting out-of- body experiences. I re-read my books on astral projection and spent many nights concentrating on the light and sound of God and waiting for the "exit" to take place. I went to extremes: I ordered a *Hemi-Sync* machine from the Monroe Institute. This is an electronic device that delivers audio tones to each ear, but frequency shifted in a manner that was thought to entrain both halves of the brain to "synchronize" with alpha, beta, theta, or delta frequencies. I thought this might help in achieving an OBE; it did not. After a year of concentrated effort, I found that I was unable to experience anything even remotely similar to astral projection. My dreams remained routine, vivid, and detailed, but the expected teacher never made his or her presence known; I was unable to leave my physical body. Not yet giving up my goal, I ordered a DreamLight from the Lucidity Institute. Dr. Stephen LaBerge, who wrote his PhD thesis on lucid dreaming, invented this electronic device. It incorporates a sleep mask with built-in light-emitting diodes whose pattern of flashing can be programmed in a variety of ways to signal the user that a dream is in progress. The light signals are strong enough to be recognized in the dream, but not enough to wake the dreamer. Unfortunately, being lucid within my dreams, as enjoyable as they were, did not help me to achieve projection of my astral body; the year passed without my reaching the astral plane; the studies of Eckankar and lucid dreaming did not accomplish the OBE task. It had been an interesting but unrewarding 12 months. As far as I was concerned, Eckankar had been a red herring; I was ready for the next assignment. An extremely important lesson was biding time, waiting for me—and not very far from home.

Chapter 5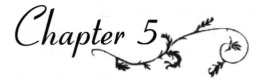

The Tree of Life

In the end, words are birds and experience is the tree they roost in. The power of inner truth is rooted in the tree. Birds come and go.

—The I Ching

In April 1984, I traveled from the Big Island to the island of Oahu to attend the annual meeting of The American Association of Neurological Surgeons (AANS). Honolulu, only a 40-minute flight from my home, had been chosen as the conference site. I was three years out of neurosurgical training and finally eligible to take the oral board examination, which would lead to certification. This would be my last academic hurdle and a final stamp of approval from my neurosurgical peers. I would then be eligible to join the AANS.

I arrived in Honolulu, checked into my hotel, and spent the evening with a few friends. The next day I found my friend, Tyrone

Hardy, an African-American neurosurgeon whom I'd first met when I traveled to New Mexico three years previously for a job interview. At the time, I was seeking a position as associate professor of neurosurgery at an academic center. I was within a month of completing my neurosurgical training and Tyrone, who served on the staff at the University Hospital, had been assigned to show me around. I regarded the city of Albuquerque as a small and inhospitable town. I imagined that were I to live there, the summer heat would be tolerable, but I had reservations about the racial climate, as it appeared to be less than welcoming to one of my complexion and integrated family profile. I quickly concluded that Albuquerque was not the place for me.

But Tyrone and I remained friends. At the beginning of our friendship, I was not aware of his high level of spiritual evolution. I only knew that he was interested in a specialized field of neurosurgery—deep brain stimulation. Now, in Honolulu, I crossed paths with him for what would turn out to be a remarkable encounter. The first day of the conference was devoted to an update on spinal cord trauma. Following the morning session, Tyrone and I spoke in the foyer of the convention center.

"Jack, what do you think about seeing the island with me?" He explained that his custom was to explore a bit and experience the flavor of the locale when he attended national meetings.

"Certainly," I said. "Let's go."

The Hawaiian term *holoholo* means to hang out or to go gallivanting; we set out to holoholo. I took along a six-pack of beer, and Tyrone agreed to do the driving, as he didn't drink. It was a perfect day, sunny and bright, and the colors of nature were magnificent. The air smelled of fresh flowers; this was paradise and for me, the beer would make it even better!

We turned onto the coastal road, when I blurted out what suddenly came to mind. "Tyrone, what do you know about astral projection?"

He was a smart guy and I wanted to check out his thoughts on the subject. There was no answer from Tyrone: he kept driving, looking straight ahead. He appeared absorbed in thought. I took a few swallows of beer and waited for his response. He turned and glanced at me, saying nothing, and then looked back to the road. Tyrone repeated this two times, which by now left me feeling rather silly at having asked such an off-the-wall question. I felt perplexed and didn't know whether to change the subject or wait for an answer. I decided to sit tight for what must surely be an insightful response; the suspense was killing me.

Another minute passed, and then he turned to me and spoke profoundly: "You should not be interested in astral projection just for the sake of *doing* it. Once you become enlightened, this and many other things will begin to happen."

Tyrone's remark stunned me and reverberated in my mind. I had asked many people about astral projection, but I'd never received a response such as this. I told him that he was correct; I had been trying for years to induce an out-of-the-body state, but had been unsuccessful. From my question, he must have sensed that I was a novice on the subject of psychic experiences. It was a stupid question to ask. I thought about his choice of words: "Once you become enlightened." I took the opportunity to run more thoughts by him, saying that I was functioning under conditions I considered stressful. He asked me to explain.

"The problem is, I'm in the middle of a divorce but I seem to have little or no control over the situation.

"And?"

"The board examination in neurosurgery is coming up and I've been too frazzled to even begin to study." I was referring to the oral exam consisting of three hours of questioning by department heads selected from various neurological and neurosurgical training programs around the country. One hour is devoted to cranial surgery, one to spinal surgery, and the final hour to neurology. It would be a difficult examination. At this time, most days were unhappy ones for me; things were not going smoothly. I summed up my thoughts and anxieties regarding my life by saying, "So you see Tyrone, I happen to be up shit's creek. In spite of my personal problems, I've _got_ to pass that exam. Do you have a paddle for me?"

No response.

We drove in silence for a few miles and then he turned into Ala Moana beach park near the shade of a large banyan tree. We parked the car and continued on foot along a sandy path toward the ocean. I kicked off my flip-flops; the sand felt good on my bare feet. Suddenly, I felt strange. The sensation was like that of an electric field surrounding me. I guess you could call it "hairs standing on end." The locals call it "chicken skin." Something was about to happen.

We continued down the path to the shoreline and sat on a large log of driftwood. Palm tree branches swayed in the wind against the backdrop of blue Hawaiian skies. The temperature had reached the 80s and the breeze from the ocean felt cool and soothing. It was then that Tyrone asked, "Are you familiar with the Tree of Life?"

"No," I said, feeling embarrassed by my ignorance.

He took a branch from a nearby tree. "Let me show you something." He drew a complicated pattern in the sand comprised of many swirls and squiggles. I was at a loss to figure out what he was doing. Before I could understand what he intended, he stopped drawing.

"You are here." He used his tree branch to mark an indentation in the sand at the top of the pattern of loops and swirls, poking it several times with the tip of his stick. "It is no longer important *how* you arrived at this point or *how long* it took you to reach it. The important thing to realize is that you have reached this point and now you're ready to go up the tree of life. Consider these as the roots of the tree." He traced a few more curvilinear lines in the sand. I had a flash of Twitchell's Tarzs: Tyrone was dark and he wore a beard!

"The particular path you took," he said as he momentarily stopped moving the stick, "is no longer relevant to your current situation. Your route might have been difficult and more demanding then another's more direct one, but the important thing for you to realize is that *now* you are *here*." With his stick he re-emphasized the area that represented the base of the tree of life. "You must move up the trunk, avoiding as many of the side branches as you can. The important experiences are found along the main stem, en route to the apex." He continued his drawing, producing a vertical line in the sand extending from the point he called the base. He then marked off six or seven side branches with short straight horizontal strokes.

"What's the significance?" I stood and began pacing the sand. My pulse quickened, and the hairs on the back my neck were now at full attention. "I told you, it is *stress*, man, things messing with me every day, and it will not stop. What does climbing an imaginary tree have to do with it?"

"Please sit," he commanded and motioned to the log. He stared at the ocean. A calming effect soon swept over me. Was that because of the beautiful scenery or because of the message now being delivered to me? Or both?

"Now," he said, "look far to the left, and tell me what you see."

I looked and noticed that there was a house in the distance. A rainsquall hovered above the house before a dark sky. "I see rain," I said. "Why?"

"I'll explain. Look way off to your right, and describe *that* scene to me."

There was a change; the ocean extended to the horizon with a few gentle whitecaps here and there; the sun shone brightly over the water. It reminded me of the first sentence in Richard Bach's *Jonathan Livingston Seagull*: "It was morning, and the new sun sparkled gold across the ripples of a gentle sea." Within that 180-degree sweep, the situation changed dramatically from one of shadow, gloom, and dampness, to one of warmth, sunshine, and peace.

"All right," he continued, "tell me something." He turned and transfixed me with his dark eyes. "How do you want your life to be? Do you want it murky," he looked to his left at the storm, "or *bright*?" He gestured toward the right. "The significance of the Tree of Life is that now that you have reached the base, you can have your life the way you want it. No longer do you have to go with the flow. That's how you got up the creek in the first place! Now you are awake and ready to take charge of the situation." With that, he snapped his fingers in my face.

I felt as if something had changed inside my body. My hearing seemed to be affected; the blue of the ocean and the sound of wind seemed to fade into oblivion as I thought about what he had said. Then, just a quickly as things had dimmed, vision and hearing returned.

Who is this guy, an angel?

"Wait a minute," I said. "Take charge? I have been trying hard to deal with the situation but problems keep piling up on me. *Take charge*? Are you kidding? I am barely able to keep treading water. I've got lawyer problems, money problems, and worse—"

"That's the point!" he interjected, jumping to his feet. "You have been *allowing* problems to control *you*. The house over there has no choice but to endure the downpour. You, on the other hand, can duck the deluge of trouble if you so choose. I am here to tell you that there is a way you can stop the pain and suffering. You simply have to wake up!"

He sat down again, curled his toes into the sand and continued: "Listen and listen carefully, Jack. Remember when I said 'once you become enlightened, out-of-the-body experiences and many other things will start to happen?'"

"Yeah, I remember that."

"Well, don't forget it." With that, he stood and began walking to the car. He motioned me to come. I now had my oar! I could feel my pulse pounding with excitement. I had just been exposed to the way to reach another dimension.

We returned to the conference center. Before saying goodnight, Tyrone asked if he might come to Hilo to spend a day with me. He wanted to see the place that I said I would never leave. I offered an invitation.

When we arrived a few days later, my friend Mike agreed to accompany us on a night in town. The way Tyrone asked us to turn down the music in the car was unusual. We were headed to a nightclub and he had offered to sit in the backseat. Mike drove, proud of his new Jeep; I sat up front.

"You're not ridin' dirty, are you Mike?" I whispered.

"Naw, man," he replied. "I know you've got a high-class guest tonight. I'm good."

Music blared from the CD player. Tyrone leaned forward and said, "Do you guys know that Aborigines can hear a conversation the length of a football field?" The way he put it was in the form of short but telling allegory. I turned the volume down; it was painful to his sensitive ears!

We had a good evening with Tyrone, and after a sound night's sleep, he returned to New Mexico. I didn't think about his Tree of Life until two weeks later when he called me. After a brief chat, the reason for his call was made clear.

"Jack, I left my Hawaiian shirt at your house. Would you be kind enough to mail it back to me? I bought it as a keepsake for the great time I had."

It is of note that in the week following Tyrone's visit, a significant event happened: the true start of my next spiritual lesson. My girlfriend at the time, Lucinda, arranged for me to get a haircut by a hairstylist that she knew. During the course of the cut and fade, the stylist spoke of an interesting sect of Buddhism where chanting held a power to alter one's life; they believed that environment and destiny could be manipulated and controlled if one followed the precise instructions written down hundreds of years ago by the Japanese Buddhist monk, Nichiren. These directives involved harnessing the pervasive forces in the universe to accomplish the task of burning off karma. The priest *Nichiren* felt that only the *Lotus Sutra* (one of many Buddhist teachings) contained the ultimate truth, and that it could be compressed into a sacred formula, which formed the words *Nam Myoho Renge Kyo*. I told Tyrone what the lady had related. His response was extraordinary!

After a few seconds of silence he said, "Get a pencil. That's where I started 17 years ago."

Seventeen years ago!?

I swallowed hard. "When you say that you *started* that long ago, do you mean—"

"Never mind that now, Jack," Tyrone interrupted. "Get a pencil, and write down what I tell you. Read *A Book of Five Rings,* by Miyamoto Musashi. Make sure that you get the translation by Victor Harris. The other translations are not as good. At first, you will think it is simply a book about sword fighting, but each time you read it you will learn something different. Musashi, having never lost a battle, ensconced himself in a cave and wrote the book. He had reached enlightenment. What you need to do now is to work on your *timing*."

I thanked him and said that I would keep in touch. Again, as when we were on the beach, Tyrone had surprised me with his perspicacity and knowledge.

The Nichiren sect was an evangelistic offshoot of *Mahayana* Buddhism. The belief was mystical and mysterious and I had been drawn to it like a bee to a flower. It amazed me to hear that Tyrone began his pursuit of metaphysical studies so many years ago. I acknowledged that I had a long road ahead. I bought *The Book of Five Rings* and quickly read it from cover to cover. That was easy; it was a small book. In the introduction, there was a photograph of a suit of samurai armor, the breastplate emblazoned with the words, *Nam Myoho Renge Kyo*. It all seemed perfectly connected and beyond coincidence: the words, the book, Buddhism, and chanting. I decided to follow Tyrone's advice and seek enlightenment as the path to the spiritual world.

Within the next few days, I completed arrangements to attend a Nichiren Buddhist meeting and asked Mike to accompany me. Strange occurrences of the Eastern variety were about to manifest for me, and they would indeed be mystical, mysterious, and an entryway to alternate methods of healing.

Chapter 6

The Power of Chanting

*Chiang spoke slowly and watched the younger gull ever so
carefully. "To fly as fast as thought, to anywhere," he said, "you
must begin by knowing that you have already arrived."*
—Richard Bach, *Jonathan Livingston Seagull*

The next evening, Michael and I drove to the meeting. We arrived to find a few dozen pairs of shoes and slippers neatly paired at the front door of the house. A Japanese woman escorted us inside to a waiting area. We heard harmonious voices emanating from the adjoining room—the occupants were hidden from our sight, but I could see the side of a large wooden cabinet located at the front of the room. This, I assumed, was the focal point. The occasional resonant sound of a gong punctuated the rhythmic chanting. Ten minutes later, the chanting stopped and we were asked to join the others in the meeting room. We passed by rows of devotees sitting in seiza (half-seated) position. They smiled and made small talk, greeting one another, while rubbing their eyes as if they had just woken up from an afternoon nap.

I now had an excellent view of the cabinet that was the center of their attention. An imposing structure, it stood more than 6 feet tall and measured half as wide. The front boasted ornately carved doors that were open to reveal a candlelit interior. Facing the cabinet (which I later learned was called a *butsudan*) was a small table that held an incense tray distributing a faint but pleasant aroma—sandalwood, as I remember it—throughout the room. A large metal bowl, perhaps 2 feet in diameter, sat to the right of the table. A strike on the bowl's rim with a padded mallet accounted for the gong sound. We were invited to inspect the inside of the butsudan. The center section held a paper scroll—a papyrus of some sort—the size of a sheet of typing paper. Inscribed on it were the Sanskrit and Japanese writings of Nichiren Dishonin. Our host explained that the vertical markings in the center of the scroll were calligraphic images representing the words Nam MyM´hM Renge KyM´, and the name Nichiren. Flanking this central inscription were instructions on the path to enlightenment. We took seats among the congregation and our host announced, "I would like to introduce Dr. Turner and his friend Michael Williams."

A polite round of applause arose among the three-dozen or so smiling faces. Several members took turns speaking of their love for Nichiren's philosophy. One woman, her hemiparesis (weakness on one side of the body) evident, delivered a moving speech. "I owe everything to the power of chanting Nam Myoho Renge Kyo. I developed a fever of 106 degrees; they thought that

I was going to die! My family and friends constantly chanted for my health. I learned how to chant and evoke the tremendous power of the Lotus Sutra to burn off karma. Slowly but surely, the fever began to decrease." At this point, she held up her contorted arm and hand. "I was left with considerable weakness, but I survived an abscess of the brain. If not for my practice of chanting, I would not be here today. There is great power in the Mystic Law. I have learned that overcoming difficulty in life is like changing poison into medicine."

She sat down to a round of enthusiastic applause. I noted the faces in the audience. During the talk, they had been attentive to her every word. She mentioned "burning off karma." She gave credit to the power of uttering the magic words, Nam Myoho Renge Kyo.

Several members now volunteered their experiences about how they chanted for health, wealth, or love. Everything they had wanted came through for them just as they had requested—only of higher quality. This was the recurring theme throughout the evening: what is asked for by chanting is even better than that which was requested. I later learned that Nam (pronounced *Naa-hm*) stems from the Sanskrit word, *namas* ("I pay homage to..."), and the words Nam Myoho Renge Kyo, when taken as a group, represent the Japanese pronunciation of the Chinese title of the Lotus Sutra. Through the practice of chanting, it was taught that enlightenment could be obtained in one lifetime.

When the speeches ended, the group turned to face the butsudan, hands prayerfully together in front of their chests. Sandalwood juzu beads were draped over their fingers. In unison, they began chanting for the better part of an hour. The session ended with three deep-throated rings of the gong. Hearing them chant for such an extended period was an intense experience. As everyone prepared to leave, I approached the cabinet. I wanted to have another look at the scroll. One of the members stopped me.

"Let me tell you about it," he said. "That rice paper, which we call the *Gohonzon*, is an exact replica of the instructions to reach enlightenment that were carved into a large piece of tree bark by Nichiren Dishonin himself. It's scaled down, of course, as the original, carefully preserved in our temple at the base of *Mount Fuji*, is more than 10 feet tall." He smiled proudly. "We have pledged our lives to protecting the Gohonzon. When we clean inside the butsudan, we hold a piece of paper or green leaf between our lips. This prevents us from blowing our tainted breath on the Gohonzon."

The scroll was the object of worship. He explained how the power of chanting had allowed him to recover from terrible illness and poverty, and that he would always be loyal to the teachings of the Great Buddha Nichiren.

The host interrupted our conversation, politely apologized for the intrusion, then took me to a small writing table. Three members were seated around the table, along with Mike. They stood—all except for Mike—and bowed politely, as was the Japanese custom, then retook their seats.

"Do you, Dr. Turner, and you Michael Williams, feel that you are ready to join Nichiren Soshu of America, which we simply refer to as NSA?" our host asked.

Mike mumbled something about how he had to "think about it." He retreated to the back of the room. I looked at the application form that had been placed before me. I knew they were eager to sign up new members, and as a physician and a respected member of the community, my joining the organization would be a feather in their cap. The principle involved was sound: tapping into powerful forces to guide one's own life and, when needed, using this energy to cure illness, poverty, and conflict. I felt that the powers they spoke of were related to my search for the spiritual world. These included the electromagnetic force, the strong and weak nuclear forces, and other even more esoteric energy fields. Nichiren taught that the "law of causality" (the relationship between cause and effect) was the principle underlying all visible and invisible phenomena and events, and that a *universal field* was responsible for the rotation of galaxies around galaxies and planets around stars. This was the power that Nichiren Buddhism tapped.

Born in the 13th century, 800 years before Einstein formulated the concept of "space-time," Nichiren had an inkling of the mysterious manner in which the universe operates. I thought about the woman with the brain infection, stroke, and eventual recovery. Had she been lucky or had she plugged into this power? Whatever the explanation, I wanted a dose of it in my life—I wanted to explore its mechanism of action. This could be another method to treat *dis*-ease.

"Absolutely," I said. I reviewed the application quickly, noting that it spelled out *diligent practice, respect, and honor for the Gohonzon.* I signed my name. Everyone clapped and stood to shake my hand.

"I'll be coming by your house with a butsudan for you!" announced one of the female members, the one who'd cut my hair the week before. In my mind's eye, I saw her delivering a large ornately carved cabinet with electrically operated doors. Tonight's event reminded me of the born-again Christian experience I'd been through a couple of years earlier, when I was cleverly persuaded to join hands and recite "The Sinner's Prayer." I'd given it a try, but with each visit to the church, the sermon left me shedding tears. The feelings of pseudo-guilt that accompanied my "rebirth" were diametrically opposite to those that I now experienced after having joined NSA. I felt empowered to correct life's problems armed with the universal laws of physics. The Gohonzon would point the way; I only needed to follow its written instructions. What could be easier than that?

After thanking our host and saying goodbye, we left, driving in silence for a while. Mike finally said, "Turner, I'll try it with you, but I don't know if I want to *join* anything." I knew it was Mike's orthodox background holding him back from fully participating in this strange, mystic practice.

"I understand, Michael. It's good that you're willing to give it a shot, brother."

When I arrived home, I looked at the materials given to me: a small booklet containing the words to five daily prayers (a mixture of Japanese kanji and Sanskrit characters). Phonetic spelling was written below each word. All five prayers were to be recited in the morning, three of them in the evening. Both sessions concluded with an extended period of *daimoku* (repeated chanting of Nam Myoho Renge Kyo). The practice was done facing the butsudan, candles lit at each side, incense burning, and the gong ready for chiming.

As promised, the woman delivered the butsudan: a small cabinet made of plain lacquered wood. My visions of a grand electrified altar evaporated in an instant. I opened the doors, and was quite surprised to find it empty!

"Excuse me," I said, "where is the Gohonzon?"

"That," she replied, "you must earn." She found a suitable place on my living room bookshelf for the cabinet. "This must be in the best room of the house, the place you would reserve for an honored guest." With that, she opened the doors of the butsudan and knelt in front of it. She took out her beads and chanted Nam Myoho Renge Kyo a few times, then turned to me and said, "When you have proven that you are serious, and that you have practiced with *true diligence*, you will be rewarded with a Gohonzon."

I got the picture—no one gets into this on a whim. That made sense. No problem. I had committed to give it a good effort twice a day for one year. She left, promising to check on my practice in the days to come.

For the next year, I went down on my knees twice a day, sat seiza with lighted candles, fresh green branches in the pots, and three sticks of incense burning. I found that the practice some-how separated mind from body during the repetitive chanting and focusing upon the scroll.

In time, the butsudan came to hold a Gohonzon, presented to me by a Buddhist priest at a private ceremony held in a stately temple in Honolulu. The Gohonzon I knelt before that day eas-ily stood 10 feet high, black (perhaps ebony wood) with gold kanji (colors I had chosen for my office). The carpet was mauve, the same as the carpet in my home recording studio! The cer-emony was surrealistic, as if a dream that incorporated bits and pieces of my real life.

I returned to Hilo that night and gave a speech to more than 200 people who gathered for the occasion. I compared the power of chanting to Einstein's famous equation, $E=mc^2$, and I explained the relationship between energy and mass. I'm a good spontaneous speaker, and for this lecture I was charged up; I had the power! The audience gave me a thunderous round of applause. I no longer had to stare into an empty altar. With the arrival of my personal Gohonzon, I had assembled all the necessary parts of the puzzle. I was determined to experience the trance-like state and produce events that would alter the environment to suit my needs.

Chanting was absolutely marvelous. Each morning, I could construct my day and decide on events that I wished to experience. Although the process did not always work in a reliable manner, for the most part it worked well. It was interesting—to say the least—to watch the events unfold just as I had requested. Furthermore, when they happened, they were delivered to me better than what I had asked for.

When I began to chant, focusing on the Sanskrit markings, I noticed that my speech soon became automatic. I could disassociate my mind from my body and become aware of remote events while continuing to utter the prayers. One session that I can clearly recall dated back to the early days when I had the empty butsudan. My mother, a child psychologist by trade, came to Hilo for a visit shortly after I joined the Nichiren organization. On that particular night, she and Mike sat outside in the hot tub. Inside the house, I chanted to the Gohonzon. As I did, I could hear their conversation clearly as if I were with them in the spa.

"Dr. Turner," Mike said, "don't think I'm going crazy too. When he told me you were coming for a visit, and you being a psychologist and all, I told him that he would have to chant by himself. He's in the house now, mumbling in Japanese to an empty box!" He snickered.

"Well Mike," she replied, "I have seen him interested in many things over the years. It's just a phase he's going through. He will soon move on to something else."

Mike said, "I want you to know that I'm *not* going to join him in going nuts." He laughed again, and even my mother began to laugh.

After finishing the session, I joined them. I told them how chanting released my mind to explore other places and other dimensions. They laughed again. I let them know that throughout my chanting and ringing of the gong, I had heard their *every word*, although the distance from the living room to the hot tub made this seem unlikely. After I reiterated their conversation verbatim, they were amazed and a bit startled to know that such a thing was possible. They stopped laughing.

I enjoyed the dissociated awareness that I achieved while chanting. It was not like the reported out-of-the-body experience, but more akin to clarity of mental processing, as in a lucid dream. The Japanese concept of *kotodama* (the power of words) implies that when words are chanted, they have a power that can change the environment. I believe that chanting sets up resonant circuits in the brain that activate usually quiescent neural pathways. I came to know this feeling of attonement quite well, and after the promised 12 months I discarded the incense sticks, the gong, and the chanting. I could recreate the feeling through meditation. Conceivably, for some, NSA's chanting could overcome personal illness and hardship, perhaps by stimulation of the immune system, through quieting the mind. However, I saw no practical way in which to use this complex and time-consuming process for the benefits of my patients. It was time for me to move on. Time to explore other methods of healing.

But, how did chanting really work? There were times when the results were as requested and that was exciting. It seemed to be truly magical. However, I came to the realization that the changes I *thought* I'd made to my environment through chanting were only parts of a script (written in the spiritual world) unfolding.

Chapter 7

The Temple in Man

*In helping others, we shall help ourselves, for whatever good
we give out completes the circle and comes back to us.*
—Flora Edwards

Near the end of my year of Buddhist chanting, I traveled to Salt Lake City to take the oral board examination in neurological surgery. The morning of the test, I took a walk around the Mormon Temple. I knew that this would be my only trip to this interesting city—or to a Mormon Temple. Tyrone told me that I now had choices: I chose to pass the test, and I did. Another of life's hurdles successfully jumped! It was not long after returning to Hilo that a strange introduction to the next level of spiritual training began. It happened when I met Gary Lyon.

One early morning, I had a moment or two before the first patient of the day. I noticed that Leilani left a note on my desk that read: *A man named Gary Lyon—never heard of him—wishes to speak to you about a music project. Yes or no? He can stop by whenever it is convenient for you.*

I looked at my appointment sheet. It was full until the lunch hour; in the afternoon I had to present a seminar on head injuries to the hospital staff. I told Lei to have him come at noon.

Gary Lyon was a polite, well-groomed handsome young man, with shoulder-length red hair. I motioned for him to sit on the couch.

"Dr. Turner, I've heard that you have a recording studio." He placed a portable tape player on my desk. "I have a project that I need to complete."

Only a handful of people knew about my recording suite. On the studio's wall, behind a massive console of mixers and tape machines, which I designed to look like a UFO's control panel, hung a stunning painting of a black lion's head with intense lava-red eyes. At the bottom of the picture was the caption, *Music has met its Master*. It was eerie: now a man named Lyon wanted to use the studio! He turned on the machine and adjusted the volume to a comfortable level. Imagine if you will for a moment, magical rites conducted in the temples and pyramid chambers of ancient Egypt; priests and priestesses gowned in religious accouterments; flame-lit chambers revealing wall paintings, hieroglyphs, and sarcophagi. Melodious tones flowed from the speakers. The music served as an ideal background for the particular setting I had just envisioned.

"This sounds professional. Who made it?" I said.

"I made it myself on a four-track recorder."

"Extraordinary," I said.

"My wife, Rosemary Clark, has illustrated a best-selling book called *The Traveler's Key to Ancient Egypt*. We're composing a slide show to promote the book. We plan to use this music."

"Gary, I'm not sure what help I can offer. Your stuff sounds great."

"Doctor, this piece needs refining. It must be *perfect*. I need access to an eight-track tape machine to do a proper mix-down. I've heard that you have the equipment and I am willing to pay for the use of your studio."

"What was the name of the book again?"

"*The Traveler's Key to Ancient Egypt*, by John Anthony West."

"So, it has to do with a key, eh? All right then, how about this?" I felt that I could trust and help him. "I rarely use the studio these days Gary. I'm either here at the office or working at the hospital. Since my divorce, I have the time to throw myself into neurosurgery." I pulled a key ring from my pocket. "You *traveled* to see me. Here is *your key*. You may use the studio at no charge."

I wish I could be there when he first sees the black lion! The studio will trip him out!

"I don't know what to say, doctor." The glow on Gary's face told the story. "Dr. Turner, we would love to have you as a guest tonight. Would you care to see our slide presentation?"

"Absolutely," I replied. We shook hands and arranged a time for the meeting.

That evening, as I parked my car in front their apartment building, I looked up to see a familiar sight. They lived across from the Pentecostal church where I had been "born again" at the start of my spiritual search. Coincidence?

Rosemary Clark, an attractive dark-haired woman in her late 20s, answered the door. She was charming, but at the same time, mystical in nature. Something about her made me think that we had met before.

"Rosemary, do I know you?"

"Indeed you do," she replied. "Your memories can be refreshed or awakened by the use of a *magic mirror*. In fact, I am working on one for you now. Care for some tea?"

This was the auspicious beginning of what would turn out to be a lasting friendship. We talked casually as Gary prepared his slide projector, amplifier, and speakers. The lights dimmed and for the next hour I enjoyed a spectacular Egyptian show of light and sound—stories of dynasties and kings; the Sphinx and pyramids; life and the afterlife. I knew I had made the correct decision to offer the use of my studio. In addition, Rosemary could teach me about something I saw in the presentation: the Egyptian concept of the *Ka* (human double or astral body), and a possible link for me to OBEs and the spiritual world.

I thanked them for the evening. I was looking forward to Gary's completion of the project and to the continued growth of our friendship. Before I left, Rosemary said, "We want to know more about your Buddhist studies. May we join you in prayer one day?"

Whoa, had I mentioned chanting to them?

"I see that you carry juzu beads." She pointed to my pocket. "I could smell the sandalwood."

This woman was sharp. So was her sense of smell!

"Why yes," I replied, "I've been studying that philosophy for the past year and—"

"Actually," said Rosemary, with a sheepish grin, "I must admit that when we heard about your studio, we also learned of your interest in NSA. We are excited about experiencing the power of chanting. In return, I'll teach you magical things about the esoteric practices of ancient Egypt."

Besides knowledge of the occult, this woman had a sense of humor!

It was my turn to sense something; I perceived the start of a new psychic adventure. I felt "chicken skin."

Gary worked diligently in the studio, completing the Egypt tape and many other projects. Rosemary introduced me to the magical traditions of ancient Egypt. The day came when they decided to leave Hilo for Honolulu, and I was saddened at their move, but at the same time grateful to have met and shared time with these interesting people.

Months later, Rosemary called with a medical question. She had developed a strange headache and a droop of her right eyelid. Her symptoms suggested the possibility of pressure on the third cranial nerve. My immediate concern was about an aneurysm (a balloon-like dilatation of an artery) or tumor close to the nerve. Diabetes can do this, but the pupil is spared.

"Do you think I have a brain tumor?" she asked.

"There may be pressure on one of the nerves that controls your eye. When you look in the mirror, is your pupil—the center part of your eye—enlarged?"

She checked, then told me, "I think it is larger than the left eye. Does that mean a brain tumor?"

"Relax. You're young to have a brain tumor, although it is part of the differential diagnosis. There are other conditions, such as vascular malformations, which could cause this problem. Contact my friend Dr. Strong in Honolulu. You need a CAT scan."

I gave her the clinic number and she promised to keep me apprised of her situation. The next day, she called to say that Dr. Strong immediately ordered a CAT scan, which showed an enhancing lesion (one that gets brighter on the film after intravenous iodine) behind her eye. They told her that this was most likely a tumor or possibly an aneurysm: a study to show blood vessels by special X-ray techniques. She was scheduled to have an angiogram.

"Doctor," she said, "will you do something for me?"

"Of course, what do you need?"

"Do you remember the book I gave to you last year, *The Temple In Man*? I'd like to have it back if you're finished; I need to check some references."

I remembered the book, written by renowned Egyptologist, René A. Schwaller de Lubicz. It described his theory of the Luxor Temple, suggesting that its architecture and layout represented the human body. Rosemary knew I would have an interest in de Lubicz's depiction of the brain. I returned the book to her and thought little more about the matter until three days later, when she called again.

"Aloha, doctor." She sounded happy. "You'll never guess what happened!"

"Is it about the angiogram?" I asked.

"Yes! I want to tell you of the extraordinary event that happened before the test. Remember the book you returned? Well, when it arrived, I didn't have time to open the package. I set it on my nightstand. That night, I awoke with a start; I heard *your* voice, doctor, just as plainly as I hear you now, *whispering* into my ear."

"Were you dreaming, Rosemary?"

"No, it was much more than that. Your words were: 'Rosemary, it is at the Transept of the Temple.' I awoke with a start and turned on the light; I noticed your package on the nightstand." There was a pause as she collected her thoughts. "I opened the wrapping, removed the book and looked in the index. I found *transeptum.*"

"And?"

"The *transept* of Luxor Temple is a representation of the *cavernous sinus* (an area of cranial nerves, venous plexus, and the internal carotid artery) of the brain, according to de Lubicz." Then she began to laugh. "When I went for the angiogram yesterday, Jack, I told them, 'I know exactly what is wrong,' and they said jokingly, 'Sure you do.' I told them that I have an aneurysm in the cavernous sinus on the right side, and they wondered how in the world I had come up with that! They called me today with the results of the study. Guess what? I have a *giant* aneurysm in the cavernous sinus!"

What serendipity! At the time she had her prophetic dream, I was studying for my oral board examination in neurosurgery. I took a month to prepare for the test. Two days before her dream, I decided to spend an entire day on aneurysms of the cavernous sinus. It was about the toughest problem a neurosurgeon could face, so I figured if I knew how to handle that, then everything else would be a walk in the park. An enlargement of the artery here—an aneurysm—would produce ptosis of the eyelid, and worse: it could rupture, resulting in sudden death. I wanted to see those X-ray films. It was then that I experienced the *second* metaphysical event connected to her case.

By what at first appeared to be coincidence, I had been scheduled to assist in surgery at the Honolulu clinic where Rosemary had her tests. I thought this would be an opportune time to view her angiogram. Only in retrospect did I realize that my being at the clinic was no accident, no coincidence—there was an important reason for me to see her films.

The radiology department put her films on an alternator (a back-lit-servo-driven mechanism) for my review. I called up Rosemary's films. There it was: a giant aneurysm of the internal carotid artery *within* the cavernous sinus. It looked like a tarantula, ominous and threatening. As I stared at it in amazement, a name came to me. I murmured aloud, "*Hosobuchi*!"

When I returned to Hilo, I looked in one of the neurosurgical texts that I had studied for the board examination. In the chapter, *Aneurysms of the Cavernous Sinus*, I found a footnote reference to Dr. Yoshio Hosobuchi, professor of neurosurgery at the University of California, San Francisco (UCSF)! It was a report of seven cases of giant aneurysms of the cavernous sinus that he had treated with cardiac bypass, hypothermia (cooling the body), and direct repair of the aneurysm within the sinus. If you open the cavernous sinus without taking these precautions, the venous plexus within the sinus may bleed uncontrollably and the aneurysm may rupture. I called Rosemary and recommended that she call Dr. Hosobuchi and ask him if he would be willing to review her films. She packaged her angiogram and express mailed the thick bundle of X-rays to California.

The following day, Rosemary received an urgent phone call from Dr. Hosobuchi. He believed that entering the cavernous sinus and ligating the base (neck) of the aneurysm was the treatment of choice. Should she elect to have the standard intracranial approach that was suggested by the clinic in Honolulu, there was an almost certain chance (in his opinion) that the aneurysm would rupture intraoperatively.

Rosemary elected to go to San Francisco. She made it through a difficult surgery. The aneurysm had been taken care of. Other than a continued drooping of her eyelid, similar to that experienced by my patient, Mrs. Ibarra, and occasional headaches that bothered her for a time, she was neurologically intact. Her mental and physical capacities were absolutely normal. She'd overcome a life-threatening event. Ancient Egypt (the love of her life) came to her aid and gave her a longer life. Was it correct to say that communication from a spirit world was responsible for her connection to Dr. Hosobuchi? Was it our connection to de Lubicz's book that did it? If indeed my spiritual body (astral or Ka) was able to travel about, I wanted to be consciously aware of it when it happened.

Dr. Strong retired from neurosurgery and left the Honolulu clinic. Shortly thereafter, I accompanied a patient from Hilo, a close friend, to Honolulu for surgery. She had asked me to assist on her case, an intracranial aneurysm. I readily agreed. It gave me a chance to work side-by-side with Dr. Strong's replacement: *Dr. Hosobuchi!*

Years later, Rosemary Clark published the first of her many books, *The Sacred Tradition in Ancient Egypt*, a scholarly tome that she thoughtfully dedicated to me.

Chapter 8

Bullet in the Brain

We all imagine ourselves the agents of our destiny, capable of determining our own fate. But have we truly any choice in when we rise, or when we fall, or does a force larger than ourselves bid us our direction? Is it evolution that takes us by the hand, does Science point our way? Or is it God who intervenes keeping us safe?

—Heroes, TV series

If a plan exists for each of us, as I suspect might be the case, is it possible to change this plan? Can we, as Nichiren asserted (and as the chanting *seemed* to confirm), consciously control what happens to us? Or is there an unalterable script, written in stone that we must follow? The groundwork to formulate a hypothesis began with an interest in the Internet, which led me to a person named Terasa. The ensuing events made me realize that a mysterious power had a hand in saving a man's life.

The Internet was in its infancy when I paid more than $400 a month in dial-up fees; a mainland connection was all that existed for Hawaii residents. The "chat rooms" were a fun way for a tyro like me to use the computer for relaxation. Getting a screen name and an AOL account was a pleasant diversion from the complexities of neurosurgery. Before long, I was in daily contact with a woman in Michigan—my first Internet friend. I remember my excitement over hearing AOL's, "You've got mail," knowing that it was my friend, Terasa Corleone, reaching out to me from across the ocean. Our interaction involved much more than chatting and flirting on line. Fate gave her an assignment: to save a young man's life…from thousands of miles away!

I met Terasa by happenstance—or so I thought. What I didn't realize until much later was that I'd been *guided* to Terasa.

During a free moment at work, on a rainy afternoon, I selected a chat room on "spirituality." I thought there may be some interesting people chatting, and reading their posts might be something to erase the monotony that I felt. While watching the various questions and comments posted, I began to follow with interest someone called *TerasaC*. She was making intelligent remarks. I wanted to meet her. I sent a "private message," starting with, "Hello!"

"Who are you?" she replied.

"My name is Dr. Turner."

"What type of doctor are you?"

"Brain surgeon."

"Sure, and I'm a rocket scientist from Detroit!"

"So am I—but from Hawaii."

It took convincing, but she soon came to realize that I was not pulling her leg. We began to chat daily.

I was between patients one Friday morning, so I logged on to the chat. My friend Terasa awaited my appearance. While we were chatting about mundane things, I took a phone call from Dr. James Ball in the emergency room.

"I've got one for you: a gunshot wound to the head; self-inflicted. I've got a tube in him (a breathing tube). His respirations are irregular and the only thing saving him is his pickled brain. I had to bust him twice (cardioversion with paddles). They found him face down on the ground, covered by his tent."

"How's that?"

"He lives in a tent. His blood alcohol level is three times the normal limit," James said. "He weighs about 140 pounds. Friends say he downed about six half-liter Canadian beers during the past two hours. Then 'bang.' It was a handgun, a .38 special."

A bullet in the brain is generally fatal. What happened in this case made me wonder if such a bullet is *fated* and only sometimes fatal. I continued to message Terasa as I listened to the doctor: "I'm getting a call now about a guy who just shot himself in the head," and, as James added more information, "he lived on the beach. His friends heard the shot—they found him on the ground with a gun in his hand. When they last saw him alive, he was drunk out of his gourd."

"What are you going to do?"

"I'll check him out soon, but as a rule I don't rush to such emergencies. If a guy wants to end his life, who am I to interfere?

Perhaps he has the right to kill himself? Maybe I should respect his decision?"

There was no immediate reply, only a pause of several seconds. Then came the response:

"Well, if I were having a bad day and you were on call, I'd be in big trouble, wouldn't I?"

I sat back and stared at Terasa's message.

She had made a poignant statement. Perhaps it was *not* his wish to end his life, but rather a terrible decision made on a bad day. Or perhaps someone else pulled the trigger? I made a quick decision.

"I'll tell you what—I'll save this guy's life, but I want a promise from you."

"Anything!"

"If I do this, Terasa, I want you to send him a card or letter daily, until he leaves the hospital."

"Agreed!"

"I'm out of here; I'll let you know what happens. PS: You had better buy a box or two of cards!"

I returned my full attention to the phone. Dr. Ball ran quickly through a list of vital signs such as blood pressure, temperature, respirations, and so forth. I interrupted him: "I'm on the way. Type and cross-match him for two units and notify the operating room that I want to cut in less than an hour."

I told my staff that I would be in surgery for the rest of the day; I was headed to the OR. How did I know that I would be in surgery? It's a sixth sense that comes with time and experience.

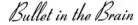

Or was it a *seventh* sense that connects with the spiritual world, resulting in *knowing?*

I wasted no time getting to the emergency room. Before this day, I'd treated the rare suicide attempt with what some would call a *laissez-faire* attitude, that is, let people do what they choose. Terasa sparked a new way of thinking: Did I have any right to decide about life and death *before seeing the patient?* Didn't a patient deserve a doctor who was willing to *rush* to his side? I pondered this issue as I entered the emergency room.

The patient (around 30 years old) was semi-comatose. He responded appropriately to painful stimuli—when pinched on his finger, he would pull away. This indicated that the stimulus was getting through to him and he was reacting correctly, which was a good sign. Another good sign: The pupils of his eyes reacted to light. Dr. Ball had performed a successful resuscitation. I examined the wound. When a bullet enters the skull, a rule of thumb is that the entrance wound will most likely be small, and if the slug leaves the cranium, the exit wound can be large. This man had a small entrance wound on the right side of his skull just above the temple. The exit wound was in the left-frontal region of the skull and was the size of a quarter.

There was no family from whom to seek surgical permission. The patient had no identification. The acquaintances that reported the gunshot lived on the beach near him. I obtained verbal permission by phone (from an on-call judge) to operate on "John Doe." This man would live.

The surgery went smoothly and I was able to debride (clean up the wound) and remove fragments of in-driven bone and bullet. By the time I finished he had been ID'ed as Lanny Mason, a fisherman.

I met Lanny's mother after the surgery. She filled in the blanks about her son's history. It was unremarkable: Lanny dropped out of society and preferred to live on the beach, keeping to himself. She began to cry softly.

"I understand. I'm sorry," I said, offering her a tissue. "So there was no question that this was a self-inflicted injury?"

"They found the gun in his hand. Two people saw him alone in his tent just before they heard the gunshot. His tent collapsed over him as he fell to the ground."

Wow! Covered up automatically in preparation for burial!

I listened intently to the mother's forthright presentation of events preceding her son's attempted suicide. Terasa was correct: the victim *did* have a "bad day." But did he want to end it all, or was his unsuccessful suicide attempt the result of alcoholic debauchery? What if someone else had shot him and placed the gun in his hand? And what if, in my ignorance (laziness, perhaps), I had decided from the office that the wound was grave and inoperable: then it would have been a *really* bad day for him.

Lanny's postoperative course was amazing. He began to respond fittingly to verbal commands such as, "Squeeze my hand," and "Open your eyes." As I made rounds that first postoperative week, Lanny's mother approached me.

"Who is this person, Terasa Corleone?" She sent this card today and as far as I know, Lanny had no friends in Detroit."

She handed me a handmade greeting that read: "Aloha Lanny! Even though you do not know me, I am praying for you Lanny, and I will pray every day for you to get well quickly."

The signature read, "A distant friend, Terasa Corleone."

"Isn't that name, Corleone, the name of a Maf—?"

"Not hardly, Mrs. Mason," I interrupted, calming her down. "Let me explain."

I related the story of my meeting Terasa to Lanny's mother. She was amazed to know that a perfect stranger would care about her son. I told her that because of Terasa, Lanny is alive.

The letters and cards from Terasa continued to arrive as promised. Lanny's mom posted each one on the wall of his room. She read them to her convalescing son. I was making rounds one day as Lanny's mother sat by her son's bedside, reading a letter to him. I listened in:

"Dear Lanny. This is the second week of your hospital stay and Dr. Turner tells me that you are able to eat and to say a few words. You will never know how proud I am of your progress. It is my hope that my husband and I will be able to travel to Hawaii and meet you in person. Please know there are folks in faraway Michigan who love you very much, and pray for your speedy recovery."

Lanny often looked at the wall and the notes from Terasa. He would stare and stare at those cards. Somebody, other than his mother, cared about him! Terasa Corleone continued to write until he left for the rehabilitation hospital. The cards and letters went with him, carefully wrapped in the shirt that he wore on the day of the injury. In time, he was able to walk without assistance and carry on a labored but fairly decent conversation. I learned years later, from a caretaker who spent time with Lanny, that he often expressed gratitude at having survived his suicide attempt. He was sorry for what he had done, and despite his residual neurological impairment, he cherished life. Amazingly, and as according to plan, that caretaker who provided this information turned out to be my girlfriend of years before—Lucinda! Terasa had guessed right; Lanny *was* having a bad day when he put the gun to his head.

This experience changed the way I approached suicide attempts. I realized that it was not my job to play God, and I must simply do what has to be done. There is a plan to everything and the best that I can do—and should do—is play my part as best as I can. Never again would I bring down the final curtain until it was *certain* that nothing further could be done. That was the message. Terasa had been the messenger.

Things fell into place for Lanny, just as if they were meticulously scripted. The timing was beyond coincidence: my "chance" meeting with TerasaC in a spirituality chat room; the call from Dr. Ball while online with Terasa; her mention of "a bad day," which spurred me to take lifesaving action; and finally, feedback from Lucinda to let me know that everything worked out in Lanny's best interest.

In retrospect, I had little choice in the matter. It was as if the plan for Lanny was composed earlier, long ago written in stone. Terasa Corleone, Dr. Ball, and I were only actors following (without being consciously aware of it) a script. I couldn't help but wonder *when* and *where* such a plan, if it existed, had been written…and by *whom*?

I was about to meet a man with the answers: Mokichi Okada.

Chapter 9

A Man of Light

It is not possible to have a reasonable belief against miracles.
—Blaise Pascal, Pensées

The busy day began in routine fashion. After making hospital rounds, I arrived at my office to find a manila envelope on my desk with a note: *Please go over these items and call Mr. Yasuo Kikuchi when finished.* My office manager told me that a ward clerk at the hospital thought that I might be interested in reviewing pamphlets and brochures concerning something "right up Dr. Turner's alley." I glanced briefly at papers about farming, The Medical Art of Japan, and some other stuff. I had no recollection of anyone named Kikuchi, and I'd never heard of the medical art of Japan. Farming held no interest. Patients were waiting. I put the package on a stack of take-home journals. Little did I know that a spiritual path was knocking at my door, and I was too busy to answer.

One week later, after performing surgery on a herniated disk, I had time to check on a postoperative patient. I stood in the vestibule outside of the operating rooms, then paused and looked to my left, then to my right. For some unfathomable reason, I debated which direction to take! What kind of nonsense was this? I was momentarily stuck in the hallway wondering which way to go. I had an inner feeling that the corridor to the right was calling, and that I would find something of great interest waiting for me.

As a heads-up alert, the powers that be must have decided that the chicken-skin sensation would be *de rigeur* for me. I was feeling it now!

I went to the right. Reaching the end of the hallway, I almost collided with my friend Katie Kosora, the surgical floor's ward clerk, as she passed through the door. She told me, "Do you know that the bones of Father Damien's hand will be in the chapel at 2:30 today, displayed in a fancy koa-wood ossuary?"

"I knew about the return of a portion of his remains to Moloka'i but that's about it."

Father Damien had established a leper colony on the northern cost of Moloka'i in 1860. The return of the bones was a huge thing for Hawaii, as this Roman Catholic priest would eventually be canonized as a saint. Catholics felt that the relics of a martyr had *mana* (power)—imbued with a spiritual energy that remained after death. The entourage escorting the bones would stop in Hilo before ending the tour on Moloka'i Island.

"Did you get the package from Mr. Kikuchi?" she asked.

"So *you're* the one who told him about me?"

She nodded and asked if I had ever heard of *moa* (pronounced "mo-ah"). In an instant I remembered that word. Several years ago during surgery, from out of the blue, a circulating nurse said, "Dr. Turner, Have you heard of the *moa* people in Hilo?

"No," I'd replied, remembering that the word means chicken in Hawaiian. Moa people? I wondered what she was trying to say.

"It's a Japanese group that heals at a distance, and M-O-A—she sounded it out by letters—as they like to say, stands for the Mokichi Okada Association."

She held the palm of her right hand toward me, explaining their belief that emitting light from the hand could cure illness. At the time, I had little interest in alternative methods of treatment. I did what I was trained to do: "Heal with Steel" (an adage that all surgeons know). Now, two years later, I heard the word *moa* for the second time.

"Is that what the package is about, Katie?"

"Yes. They asked me if I knew of any doctors who they might talk to about researching their work. I told them to contact you. It's destiny at work—you like weird stuff!"

"I'm interested. Tell your friend Mr. Kikuchi that I'll review the materials and get back to him soon."

Good thing I took the passageway on the right. Had I gone the other way I would have missed her. The package from Mr. Kikuchi might have sat untouched.

After work, I returned home to find my friend, Dr. Ed "Tick" Briscoe waiting for me. The nickname of Tick had been given to him because of the peculiar way that he frequently blinked his blue-gray eyes. He was a blend of American Indian and African American; I felt that this put him in tune with psychic phenomena. I thought it prudent to ask Tick to lend his thoughts to the contents of the MOA package. I offered Briscoe tea, using the silver service my wife had recently polished, setting the contents of the package on the tray.

We began our investigation. The first pamphlet described *Nature Farming* and the use of "green manure" (such as clover or grass) for fertilizer, rather than animal excrement. We read articles on methods of eliminating pesticides in order to grow healthy, non-polluted produce. Nature Farming, they said, relieves the body from having to deal with exogenous toxins.

"Less work for the liver and kidneys," Tick said as he scanned the pamphlet. His background in anesthesia and family practice allowed him to expound on a case of lindane poisoning (an agricultural pesticide). Lindane had recently taken the blame for contamination of locally grown papaya. We then examined a booklet about Dr. Kazuo Nitta's experience with Okada's teachings. When Dr. Nitta heard of *Johrei* (which means "uplifting of the spirit"), he was skeptical. He surreptitiously joined the organization, planning to expose Johrei as a trick and Mokichi Okada as a charlatan. Much to his surprise, he found that by using Okada's techniques, he could facilitate healing in his patients! He became deeply involved with Okada and soon advanced to the position of director of the MOA clinic in Tokyo.

"Check this out." I withdrew the next booklet, *A Man of Light.* Together, we read about Mokichi Okada, who was born in 1882. As a youth, he suffered with what his doctors called an incurable form of tuberculosis. He was an accomplished artist. While looking through an art book on fruits and vegetables (during a period when he was confined to bed), it occurred to him that if food were grown without animal fertilizers and chemical pesticides, their naturalness would have tremendous healing properties. He began to experiment in his Tokyo garden. Eventually his decision to add naturally-grown foods to his diet improved his health and that of his family. His doctors were flabbergasted; the tuberculosis had been purged from his body!

But tuberculosis was just the beginning. Okada suffered from eye disease, giving him double vision and impairing his ability to paint pictures. A subsequent injury to his hand thwarted his plans to manufacture laquerware; he couldn't control the wheel that spun the gold and silver powder. And if that wasn't enough to test his mettle, he also had to deal with poverty (bankruptcy) as well as personal tragedy (the loss of a wife during childbirth). He wanted to know *why* he had to suffer. He sought the answer in the "invisible spiritual world."

Hot dog! I was on to something. This is just what the doctor ordered! We continued to read about Mokichi Okada.

After many metaphysical experiences, a four-centimeter sphere of spiritual light energy mysteriously lodged within his abdomen, and later became a place of residence for the spirit of the *bodhisattva, Kannon.* Okada found that this energy, when coupled with a natural food diet and the appreciation of art and beauty, could not only cure illness, but also poverty and conflict.

The next booklet in the stack described a lecture given by Ilya Prigogine (Belgian chemist and Nobel prizewinner), entitled "The Converging of Western and Eastern Viewpoints on Science and Nature." Prigogine referred to the work of Dr. Raymond Moody on near-death experiences, the philosophy of the Buddhist priest Nichiren, and the views of Dr. Stephen Hawking on predetermination, all of which were subjects that held my interest.

More chicken skin.

A thin booklet described how Johrei worked. MOA members wore an amulet. Sealed inside was the kanji for light (*hikari*).

光

Hikari

It was taught that the energy residing in his abdominal cavity traveled down his arm, through the calligraphy brush, and incorporated with the ink molecules. Devotees believed that to wear this amulet linked them by *spiritual cords* to Okada and enabled them to transmit rays of spiritual light energy directly from Okada himself. Interestingly enough, Mr. Okada died in 1955.

116

As open as I was to unusual concepts, that was a difficult pill to swallow. The energy they channeled came from the spiritual world! This was similar to Reiki, a practice of healing with universal energy, which was an easier notion for me to understand. Both Tick and I had seen *Reiki* performed and we knew that the universal force did the healing work. But Johrei was different. It was Okada who, in his many books, directed where the energy was needed to treat a plethora of diseases. He described "key points" where energy should be directed. Living in Hawaii, we knew about spiritual cords. In Hawaiian mysticism, they are called *aka* cords, etheric links tying humans together; a linking of the "lower self" to the "higher self," with the strongest bonds being between blood relatives. The vital forces, as well as thought waveforms, travel by means of aka cords to establish telepathic communication. Okada's theory on spiritual cords made sense to us. It was amazing to think that here, in my hands, was the continuation of my spiritual training—literally handed to me on a silver platter!

"I don't know," Tick mumbled. "Flower power? Light from the hand?" He needed help to understand. I retrieved two books from my bookshelf: *The Secret Life of Plants* and *Into the Light*.

"Did you know that *all* of the cells of our bodies emit ultraviolet light and that photoluminescence—treating blood with ultraviolet light—was once used to cure disease?"

"Nope," he said.

"Furthermore, plants and flowers *also* emit light in the ultraviolet range."

I handed the books to him. He took them reluctantly, but soon became engrossed in a chapter on light emission from nerve cells. I waited and watched as he pulled more brochures out of the envelope. His attention was drawn to photos of artwork that Okada had collected throughout the years. There were pictorial descriptions of the museums and "healing grounds" in Hakone and Atami, Japan.

"Art, beauty, and flower arranging are important in healing," Tick said. "And, there's a chapter in your *Secret Life of Plants* book that says flowers, fruits, and vegetables emit light in the ultraviolet range."

"Briscoe, listen up. All of the cells of our bodies emit light—not just the nerve cells—and most of it is in the ultraviolet range. It is interesting to note that visible light is also emitted; single-photon detectors are sensitive enough to detect it."

"Yeah, I knew that." But he was probably telling a lie. As far as I knew, he had no interest in the physics of light emanation. Tick was a right-brained kind of a guy. "But I'm more interested in art," he continued, as if reading my mind. "Okada wanted to expose people to great works of art to uplift their spirits and facilitate healing. It says here that he became so knowledgeable about art, the dealers couldn't pull the wool over his eyes. In time, he amassed quite a collection."

He opened the leaflet to the picture of a Rodin sculpture. I wondered how exposure to truly great artwork would "uplift the spirit." Perhaps great works of art exuded a waveform that some-how interacted with the human mind (as opposed to shoddy works of art). I had heard and read enough. I called Mr. Kikuchi to arrange a meeting.

The next Friday, I headed south on the ocean highway. I turned off at the location marked on the map and drove along the steep road to its end, where I faced a straw-roofed house that clung to the side of the cliff. After parking, I was greeted by a large, barking dog; luckily, I saw that he was chained to the end of the porch. I walked up to the door, where a white-haired Japanese woman emerged and said, "Konnichiwa, Turner Sensei, Kikuchi-san ni au tsumori desu ka?"

I answered "*Hai* (yes)," although I didn't understand exactly what she said.

She bowed and ushered me inside. I removed my shoes and placed them on the *tatami* mat near the entryway. The house's commonplace facade gave no hint of the opulence within. A multi-angled skylight lit a *Koi* pond, where large, multicolored fish swam languidly. A small fountain bubbled quietly, spilling into the pond.

"*Dôzo…dôzo,*" she said, motioning me into the sunken living room. "*Syousestu wo yomimasu ka?*" I could catch her meaning this time. She asked if I were a reader of books. I understood some Japanese phrases and could speak a few myself.

"*Syousetsu wo kaku tsumori desu,*" I answered with a bow, telling her that I planned to *write* a book. She seated me by a low koa-wood table and left the room.

My attention was drawn to a framed calligraphy scroll above the fireplace mantle, which was an English translation of the

Zengen Sanji Prayer, written by Mokichi Okada. As it appeared I might be waiting for a few minutes, I got up to read it. The prayer described an ideal world of peace and harmony. Reading through it uplifted my spirit. The last few lines summarized the entire piece:

We will all enjoy prosperity, blessed with good health so we will live long.

And we will do good deeds, helping others and accumulating virtue.

Oh God, please bless us with thy great love and boundless benevolence, and help us to live in accord with thy will oparadise on earth may become a reality. As we kneel in deep reverence to pray, we pledge that we will follow thy will from our innermost hearts.

Miroku Omikami (Great God of Light), protect us and bless us with supreme happiness.

A small plaque below the prayer read: "This is to be chanted daily, without fail and with utmost sincerity."

The living room contained many *objets d' art* and I took time to scrutinize one of them, a woodblock print depicting Miyamoto Musashi, the great samurai, jumping from a rowboat, brandishing a wooden oar. Tyrone had urged me to read Musashi's book. Another coincidence?

"Turner-sensei?" The voice belonged to a diminutive Japanese man wearing a *hakama* (a wide skirt with seven pleats representing seven samurai virtues) over a *kimono*; he carried implements for making tea.

"May I offer you a drink of fine Japanese green tea?" He placed the tray on a small stand.

"Of course," I said, taking a seat opposite him in front of the table.

"It would be my assumption that as a doctor, you are familiar with the tumor-growth inhibitor in green tea? And the fact that green tea lowers blood sugar and cholesterol?"

"Not really," I replied.

"Green tea is one of five varieties of tea. And, quoting from *Qigong* master Ken Cohen, 'Green tea has an amino acid that calms the mind: drinking tea is meditation.' Do you know sensei Cohen?"

"I'm afraid that I don't know him, but his name rings a bell."

"Physicians refer patients to him for energy treatment. He may be coming to Hawaii for a workshop. You *must* make an effort to attend."

I watched with interest as he prepared the tea, beginning with a precise folding of a silk scarf or *fukusa,* which he then tucked under his belt. He filled the tea bowl with hot water, used the whisk briefly, and then emptied the water into a waste container. He cleaned the bowl with a small linen cloth, then prepared two scoops of powdered green tea and placed them gently into the bowl. As he added hot water to the brew, the sound of a *koto* waifted into the room.

"My wife loves to play. Seventeen strings!" With a brisk motion, he whipped the liquid into a frothy mixture and ceremoniously offered the bowl to me. I drank the tea in three easy swallows.

"Dr. Turner," Mr. Kikuchi said, "I have much to discuss with you." He launched into a review of Mr. Okada's background and the development of Johrei (initially called *Okada finger-pressure technique*). As evening turned to night, I found myself under Mr. Kikuchi's spell. I listened to his stories about Okada's life in Japan. Although Okada had never traveled to Hawaii, he predicted that "East would meet West" (combining the best of both worlds for holistic treatment of the patient) and it would begin in Hawaii. As far as enlightenment, Okada was truly enlightened. He was the recipient of a "4-centimeter sphere of light," which he called a gift from God, that lodged within his abdomen. On small bits of paper, he wrote the kanji character for light with an ink pen. He distributed these as the *o-hikari* amulet. By wearing this talisman, one could connect to Mr. Okada by the spiritual cords mentioned earlier, and to emit *his* healing light energy from the palm of the hand. As a scientist and physician, I wanted to learn as much as I could about it. The evening's visit ended and I thanked the Kikuchis for their hospitality, promising them that I would study Okada's philosophy.

During the next month, I studied Okada's writings. It paid off handsomely when Mr. Kikuchi stopped by my office to extend an invitation to visit the MOA center on Oahu.

"I will make it so—for tomorrow," Mr. Kikuchi said. "Mr. Alton Higaki will meet your plane."

That evening, Alton called to confirm the time of my arrival. He said that a doctor from Kona, Ray Rosenthal, would be there to receive his o-hikari amulet, and he suggested that because I was well informed about the workings of Johrei, I should also receive one.

"We wear ours all the time," he said, "even when we shower. It is made of a synthetic material, a high-tech ceramic, and will not scratch. Not only does it link us to Mr. Okada, but it serves to protect us from evil."

"Good," I said. "I'd like that."

I was on a roll now!

In Honolulu, Alton drove me to the Pacific Cultural Center. I met Mr. Ogata, the director of MOA Hawaii. After a tour of the facilities, I was escorted to a conference table where several Japanese men were waiting. Mr. Ogata asked me what I knew about the philosophy of Mr. Okada. I said that I agreed with the concepts. The practice of Nature Farming was a no-brainer for me, and the incorporation of art and flowers was easy to understand, but being a channel for the spiritual energy of Mr. Okada...well, that was something I wanted to experience for myself. I told him that my 20-year involvement with the practice of medicine, coupled with my recent interest in the workings of the spiritual world, placed me in a perfect position to embark on the study and practice of Johrei. I concluded with what I thought to be a politically correct statement: "What else, other than the gift of health, could make people truly happy? Contact with the invisible spiritual world would make *me* happy. I feel blessed to be entering a new phase of learning, a higher level of spiritual evolution." This generated a murmur throughout the room, and I could only hope (Japanese muttering not being my specialty) that it represented positive acceptance of my comments.

At that point, Dr. Rosenthal arrived. We were asked to stand facing Mr. Ogata, who then turned toward a large framed calligraphy, *The Great Divine Light*. Mr. Ogata lifted his hands to head level and clapped three times. Those assembled began a sonorous chant in Japanese, its purpose to inform Mr. Okada (who, as I said, had died in 1955) that two new adherents were about to receive their o-hikari amulets. It was their way of asking Okada for permission to continue. The monotonic chanting ended with another three claps. We received our amulets, each an inch in diameter and extremely thin. We placed them around our necks, received congratulations from those present, then went downstairs for the start of the Johrei clinic.

Two women were taking blood pressures and filling out information sheets for the clients. In the adjoining room, several hardback chairs were placed in a row; in front of each was a stool. Patients, seated on the stools, received Johrei from practitioners seated in the chairs. Alton asked me to give him Johrei and took a seat. He gave a brief explanation on the proper hand position. He directed me to visualize a beam of *spiritual light energy* radiating from my hand and penetrating his body.

I spent the next 30 minutes focusing Okada's energy on Alton's shoulders and low back. He began to sweat, even though the breeze from the window should have been cooling him. He thought it was exceptional for a first-time channeler to be able to produce such sensations of heat.

This had been an extraordinary day. I was ready to engage in a spiritual-medical practice. The previous night, I dreamt about giving Johrei with my palm outstretched. Now, I was enacting this dream. I knew that with Mokichi Okada's help, I was about to witness miracles. I had no idea that I was about to follow a meandering pathway that would manifest dramatic results with alternative methods of healing and the use of universal energy.

Chapter 10

Mr. Sugitan's Christmas

The insight to see possible new paths, the courage to try them, the judgment to measure results—theses are the qualities of a leader.

—Mary Parker Follett

I made good on my commitment to study Johrei. My Friday afternoons, formerly used for relaxation, now provided time for me to work with the MOA practitioners. I scheduled a dozen people to come each week for flower arranging and Johrei treatment. I kept accurate records of each patient's complaints and the results of our therapy. I gave several lectures on the results of combining Johrei with Western medicine. The subject matter ran the full gamut of disease entities that a neurosurgeon sees: brain injuries, brain tumors, spinal pain, pinched nerves, and headache. MOA provided cameras for *Kirlian* photography (a high-frequency/high-voltage imaging technique). I used them to record images of the hand and fingertips, before and after Johrei.

My first use of Johrei in a surgical patient was in the case of Mr. Sugitan. He was an answer to my request for something challenging with which to test Johrei, the medical art of Japan.

The Mokichi Okada Association arranged for me to tour the MOA "zones" in Japan. Mr. Kikuchi escorted me on a tour that stretched from Tokyo to Kumamoto. Four days were earmarked for visits to Okada's healing grounds and art museums in Hakone and Atami.

On December 22, 1995, I stood in the library of the *Kanzantei*, the home that Mr. Okada built in Hakone. As Mr. Kikuchi described Okada's writings on religion, philosophy, politics, and poetry, I gazed out the window at the panoramic view that greeted Okada. The splendor of *Mount Myojo* ("morning star") provided a gorgeous backdrop to the healing grounds where Okada asked his followers to place every rock and tree according to a plan that came to him from God. This was another sign. Mt. Myojo (pronounced the same as the "myoho" in the Nichiren chant) acted as a guiding light. It was clear what I must do. I made a mental agreement with whatever god or force that was listening in. I sent a silent request into the etheric realms (in a manner similar to the prayer I offered up on Mrs. Ibarra's behalf), agreeing to accept the fact that Mokichi Okada received a sphere of light that allowed him to treat illness. I promised not to question the premise that through the o-hikari amulet, this energy could be channeled. I would not be a doubter; I would *believe*. I promised to add Johrei to my medical-surgical tools. However, I asked for two things in return: First, I wanted to go back to Hilo and try Johrei on difficult and challenging cases. Second, because Okada had been willing to put in the elbow grease to become spiritually enlightened, then I was willing to give the same effort. If these wishes will be granted, then I am ready to put Johrei into practice.

I arrived in Hilo on Christmas day. The next day, at the hospital, Dr. Sam deSilva approached me, waving CT films as he came my way.

"Jack, am I ever glad that you are back! I have a patient with a large brain hemorrhage and every neurosurgeon I called on Oahu refused him in transfer. He has Xmas Disease and on top of that, he's on Coumadin (an oral blood thinner) for A-fib (atrial fibrillation—a potentially serious cardiac arrhythmia if untreated). He's comatose." He held up the scan to the light. I saw a gigantic left-parietal hemorrhage with mass effect and ventricular shift indicating high pressure.

I had heard of Xmas Disease (a type of hemophilia) as a medical student, but hadn't seen an actual case. "I have the answer for you, Sammy. We can blend Eastern and Western medicine and treat the patient with the best of both. I've just returned from Japan; I know how to do it."

This surprised Dr. deSilva. "I have no idea what you're talking about, but would you be willing to talk to the family about it?"

"Of course," I replied.

The timing couldn't have been better, as I had pamphlets on Johrei in my briefcase! Several family members looked up expectantly as we entered the ICU waiting room.

Sammy introduced me to Mrs. Sugitan, and I launched into a brief history of Mokichi Okada, Johrei, flowers, and natural foods. I informed the family that standard Western treatment would include clotting factor replacement from Honolulu, vitamin K infusion, and transfusions of fresh frozen plasma, these being the items needed to reverse the effects of the blood thinner. I told them that correcting the bleeding problems may take two or three days, but meanwhile, anti-seizure drugs, steroids, and body cooling might hold him until it was safe for me to operate and remove the hematoma. This was a lot for them to digest. As they pondered my remarks, I distributed the pamphlets.

"By combining Eastern and Western medicine, we can do our best for Mr. Sugitan. It will be my goal to afford him a chance to continue life in the best possible way. I am assuming that he is right-handed, so the injury to the left side of his brain involves his right arm and leg as well as the areas for speech—both for understanding what is said, and the ability to speak. He may not regain these functions."

"Dr. Turner," Mrs. Sugitan said, "he *is* right-handed as you say. However, I don't know much about Eastern medicine. As Seventh-day Adventists, we do believe in faith healing. But you say that Mr. Okada believed that his techniques represent a 'religion above religion,' and they are not based on faith? I'm afraid that I am a bit confused. Could you explain?"

"Certainly, Mrs. Sugitan. What Mr. Okada meant to imply was that it is a matter of transmitting his God-given gift of light. It does not depend on the patient's faith or a belief in Johrei. Okada outlined key points of the body to treat for various disease processes. It is a matter of channeling Okada's light to your husband." I showed them my o-hikari amulet and gave them a rundown on the spiritual cords that link to Okada. "In addition, it will be of utmost importance to have a fresh flower arrangement at bedside. This is something that we can do immediately."

"But the hospital told us that we could not bring flowers into the ICU."

"I understand that this is the general rule, but rules can be changed. I'll speak to the nurses. I'm certain that they will allow us to provide flowers and Johrei."

This was some heavy stuff to lay on anybody, especially a family who believed in the power of prayer, but had no inkling about spiritual light energy. Dr. deSilva looked astonished as I explained the "channeling" of energy from a person long deceased. Would they think I was off my rocker? It was time to find out.

"One floral arrangement," I continued, "is all that will be required, and in the pamphlet you will read about the healing effects of flowers." At this point I didn't launch into a discourse on the ultraviolet light emitted by flowers, plants, and vegetables— they had a lot on their plate as it was. "Would you like for me to treat your husband?"

"We want to have him with us for as long as possible. I would like you to handle it. Please save him, Dr. Turner!"

I began by examining the patient. I'd outlined everything for the family, but I had yet to see the patient or his chart. His scan showed the large clot in the left side of his brain. Printed below was the diagnosis: *Hemorrhage due to Xmas disease and Coumadin.* I used to feel guilty about using the truncated word "Xmas" instead of "Christmas." Xmas Disease (hemophilia B) came about as a result of Stephen Christmas, a five-year-old British boy who developed a bleeding disorder and was the first patient diagnosed with hemophilia type B. There are three types of hemophilia: classic hemophilia (type A), represents 85 percent of cases; type B represents part of the remaining 15 percent; and type C is the rarest of the bunch. In Mr. Sugitan's case, the missing blood protein needed for clotting—Factor IX (Christmas factor)—is derived from donors by special laboratory techniques. We would have to obtain the factor IX concentrate from Honolulu.

But lack of clotting factor IX was not the only cause of his bleeding. There had been further disruption to Mr. Sugitan's clotting system due to the drug Coumadin. Chronic atrial fibrillation, a fluttering of the chambers of the heart, could lead to emboli (small blood clots) thrown from the heart to the brain. Coumadin (an anticoagulant) was the most powerful way to thin the blood and prevent emboli; Aspirin is not nearly potent enough. Mr. Sugitan's laboratory numbers showed that he was far beyond the upper limits of safe anticoagulation. He was in the range where people start to bleed spontaneously. Only infusions of fresh frozen plasma, vitamin K, and factor IX concentrate could bring the lab numbers down to a point where I could safely perform a craniotomy and remove the clot. Any attempt to operate now would cause him to bleed to death. I had to keep him alive until then. And if I could operate, perhaps I could save him.

I told the head ICU nurse, "Will you assemble your staff in the conference room? I want to outline a new form of treatment, a non-touch energy treatment called Johrei. Also, I want to put fresh flowers in Mr. Sugitan's room and I would like permission for non-family members to visit—to administer energy treatments at the bedside."

In surgery or on the hospital floors, the surgeon is the captain of the ship. In Hilo, I had no opposition or resistance to my wishes. I was free to do what I thought best for my patients.

"We'll be happy to discuss that with you, Dr. Turner," the nurse said. "I'll be back momentarily."

Mr. Sugitan, a large Filipino man, lay comatose and attached to the usual assortment of intravenous lines and life support equipment. His pupils were mid-position and reactive to light, and he was triggering the respirator. He showed little spontaneous movement of his right arm and leg; his left arm required restraints to prevent him from reaching for the endotracheal tube and the intravenous lines. His chart revealed that his clotting times were sky high as Dr. DeSilva had remarked. Hopefully, they would not take too much time to correct.

"We're ready, doctor," the nurse said. I followed her to the conference room and spoke with the staff, explained Johrei, and how I planned to treat Mr. Sugitan. I requested permission for a floral arrangement to be maintained in his cubicle and for MOA members to come daily to channel Johrei. I gave them a more detailed, technical talk than I'd given to the family. They unanimously agreed to follow my recommendations, noting that they would convey their approval to the hospital administrator. They knew that I have always gone to bat for the patient, and if I felt this was the way to treat Mr. Sugitan, then they would back me up. Also, this was Hawaii, where the attitudes are not inflexible—people are open to new ideas. I would have had a great battle at most mainland hospitals by the mere suggestion of such a radical approach. But I was not planning to use Johrei and flowers as alternatives to standard treatment. In this case, Johrei would be complementary; I planned to operate on Mr. Sugitan.

And so it began—fresh flowers at the bedside, a Johrei channeler arriving daily from MOA, and the requisite infusions and injections of medications, steroids, anticonvulsants, and blood supplements. The patient held his own, and three days later I took him to surgery. By means of a large craniotomy, I removed the hemorrhage from the left side of his brain. After placing the last suture, I gave him 20 minutes of intraoperative Johrei, letting Okada's light flow through a spiritual cord to me, and then to the patient. This was a first for Hawaii and perhaps for any medical center (and surely for any neurosurgical operating room) outside of Japan.

His recovery was spectacular, and despite the odds against him, he not only made it through the procedure, but also the difficult postoperative period involving several days of induced coma with barbiturates, forced hyperventilation, and total-body cooling. Within two weeks, he could sit in a chair and feed himself with his left hand—the right arm remaining paralyzed and nonfunctional. He could not speak clearly, but he could understand what was said to him and when sitting in the hallway, securely strapped into his wheelchair, he smiled cheerfully to the passersby as he sat eating his meals, happy to be alive.

During his post-operative recovery, Mr. Sugitan developed gastric bleeding, first noticed as bright red blood in his bowel movements—another life-threatening problem. We treated this with antacids, blood transfusions, and intense Johrei. The bleeding stopped. This condition alone could have been fatal, but he made it through. I wrote his discharge four weeks after surgery to the care of his family. Their wish had been granted: they had him back.

Shortly after his discharge, Mr. Sugitan's oldest son asked to speak with me about his father. "Dr. Turner, we appreciate all that was done for my dad—by you and the entire hospital staff. He's with us again, and we cherish every moment. Thank you!"

"You're welcome, though it was not I who saved your father, but forces far superior in nature to my abilities."

"And that's what I want to speak with you about. I have something to say that you'll find interesting. Dr. Turner, I'm a pump technician for cardiac surgery in Honolulu and, for the most part, a technically minded guy. I don't claim to know much about the spirit world and things like that, but I want to say that during the time he had the gastric bleed, and Mr. Kikuchi came daily to administer Johrei…" He stopped short, embarrassed with what he was about to say. I urged him to continue. "Well doctor, even though the blinds were usually closed and not allowing much light into the room, as my brother and I watched Mr. Kikuchi treat dad with his outstretched palm…well, we wanted to tell you that…we *saw* something!" He was having great difficulty speaking. I wondered what had been so startling for the Sugitan brothers. "We're sure that it was not a trick of light and shadows; we are certain that we saw traces of light extending from Mr. Kikuchi's hand, reaching out to my father."

I could only think to say, "*Is that so?*"

"Yes. We thought that you would like to know. It kinda tripped us out!"

I thanked the young man for coming forward with the information. I knew from my studies that most of the light emitted by the human body is in the ultraviolet range but, as I had told Dr. Briscoe, a small portion is in the visible range. The majority of this light (according to scientific studies) is emitted from the fingertips and, surprisingly, from the fingernails. It was great to hear confirmation like this from family members. I found it hard to describe my feelings at that moment. It seemed like the son's revelation was a sign that indeed, I was on the right path— a blend of Eastern and Western medicine to holistically treat patients.

In the months that followed, many interested parties, doctors and nurses alike, approached me to explain how flowers and Johrei had facilitated Mr. Sugitan's recovery. After a lecture that I gave at Hilo Medical Center, a surprising number of medical practitioners became involved in Johrei, the medical art of Japan. My wish had come true. Mr. Sugitan had been an extremely difficult case. But was this a convincing enough demonstration?

Unbeknownst to me, waiting in the wings was a case where not only had all hope been abandoned for the patient, but his family had been told that he was—for all intents and purposes— dead!

Chapter 11

Called to Say
I Love You

Whenever Richard Cory went downtown,
We people on the pavement looked at him.
He was a gentleman from sole to crown,
Clean favored, and imperially slim.

And he was always quietly arrayed,
And he was always human when he talked.
But still he fluttered pulses when he said,
"Good morning," and he glittered when he walked.

So on we worked, and waited for the light,
And went without the meat, and cursed the bread;
And Richard Cory, one calm summer night,
Went home and put a bullet through his head.
    —From Edwin Arlington Robinson's, *Richard Cory*

I was living my dream of blending Eastern and Western medicine in my neurosurgical practice. The hospital staff got in the swing of things. They allowed fresh flowers at the patients' bedsides; they had no objection to Johrei practitioners giving treatments; they lauded the incorporation of natural foods into the hospital diets. The result of Mr. Sugitan's treatment indicated that perhaps I had connected with Okada's invisible spiritual world. I wanted to continue my investigation of Johrei to prove to myself that it was *not* an illusion, and that complementary medical practice was superior to conventional medicine alone. Although Mr. Sugitan's recovery was amazing, a truly astounding case was that of young Daryl Ueno—the boy with the handsome face.

One Monday morning I ran into Dr. Glenn Akiona, an anesthesiologist, in the hospital parking lot. He said, "Hey, did you see that kid with the gunshot wound to the head yesterday?"

"What kid?" I asked.

"I didn't see him, just heard about him. Apparently it was pretty bad."

"I wasn't on call yesterday, but if there was something that could have been done, they would've called me."

"I understand he's still in the ICU with his head wrapped in chucks (disposable bed pads) and left for dead."

"Well, I guess that's it for him. I'm on my way to do a herniated disc."

After the routine surgery I changed clothes and started to leave for my downtown office when I heard my name being paged to the ICU. Strange, I thought, because I had no patients there. Then it came to me—this probably involved the gunshot incident Glenn had mentioned earlier. I called the ICU and sure enough, a consultation had been requested on the boy.

"What's his name?" I asked the nurse. "I'll stop by radiology and pick up his scan."

"Ueno," she replied, "Daryl Ueno. The family said that you know him."

The name didn't sound familiar. I had seen so many patients that I'd given up trying to remember them by name.

I entered the X-ray department and pulled the patient's folder. The first sets of films were CT scans of the lumbar spine. I looked at the identification tag on the film sheets and saw my name as the ordering physician. That scan was normal, but his head scan told a tragic story—a portion of the left skull was missing and there were numerous bullet fragments in the brain. I left for the intensive care unit.

A clerk guided me to cubicle 4B, saying, "I hope you can help the boy—he's so young."

An endotracheal tube protruded from the patient's mouth; his head was wrapped in paper towels. I didn't recognize him. Seated at the bedside was a young girl, sobbing quietly; a woman stood next to the girl, her back to me. An eerie stillness pervaded the room.

"Excuse me," I said. The woman turned toward me. It was Daryl's mother. I remembered her; she lived in my neighborhood. Now it came back to me. I met Daryl years ago following a basketball injury that resulted in a strain of his back. I saw him again after a hammer struck him during a fight. I examined him in the ER, sutured his laceration, and sent him home with a head sheet and a reminder to always do the right thing. Now, years later, fate had once again delivered young Daryl into my hands. The first time I treated him had been trivial; the second had been bad; this time, however, was far worse. The Japanese have a saying: "Sandome no shojiki," meaning that the truth comes out the third time around, or more simply, "Third time lucky." Daryl and I were together again—for the third time.

Daryl's mother said, "We were told yesterday that he was brain dead and that I should consider donating his kidneys and liver. But his girlfriend," she nodded in the direction of the distraught girl, "remembered him say many times that if he was ever injured critically, he did *not* want to be an organ donor. His step-father is flying back from California. We want to stay with Daryl until the end."

I motioned for her to accompany me to the nursing station. "I understand," I replied, leafing through his chart for more information on his condition.

"The doctors called Honolulu and were told that nothing could be done. A neurologist saw him last night and had the same opinion. I agreed to discontinue the respirator. We are waiting for him to take his last breath. When I heard that you were in the hospital, I wanted you to see him. You helped him so much in the past."

As we sat down at the desk, I put Daryl's CT scan on the view box. I wanted to say the right thing to this devoted mother.

"As you know ma'am, Daryl has what appears to be a fatal insult to his brain. I understand that his girlfriend heard the shot and found him on the floor yesterday morning, the gun, a .357 Magnum, in his hand. Is that correct?"

"Yes, he was upset. He lost his best friend in a hunting accident, and his car stereo business was floundering. He had filed for bankruptcy."

"Take a look at this area," I said, pointing to the scan image where the bullet entered. "This means that even if Daryl survived the injury, he would probably be unable to use his left arm and leg. You know him; would he want to live that way?"

"No," she said grimly. "He would not want that. But there is something I don't understand. He respond to *me*?"

"Responds to *you*? What do you mean?"

Tears ran down her cheek. "Well, doctor, he'll squeeze my hand when I ask him."

Hold on a second. Nobody who is close to being brain dead is going to follow commands!

"Explain," I commanded Mrs. Ueno.

"When I held his hand earlier today, from time to time, I could feel him giving me little squeezes. Then, each time I requested him to squeeze, he would."

My mind boggled at her words. "This might change everything," I said, barely able to hide my excitement. "Let me examine him."

I took a second look at Daryl. His breathing was shallow, but regular. This was a good sign. His pupils were not dilated, nor were they pinpoint in size; they were mid-position and reacted to light, also a good sign. In fact, both indicators meant that he was not brain dead. He was flaccid—after lifting his arm or leg and letting go, the extremity would flop back to the mattress. Next, I administered the most important part of my examination. I placed two fingers from my right hand into his right hand and leaned over the bedrail to within an inch of his ear. "Daryl, squeeze my hand." I was rewarded with a weak, but definite squeeze. Yes, he *had* squeezed my hand! "Now let go!" I commanded. At once he released it. I was amazed at Daryl's response, and asked him to repeat this maneuver. He responded appropriately. "Now," I said, my mouth still close to his ear, "open...your...eyes!" Slowly, his eyes opened to meet my gaze, and then gradually closed. This was a repeatable response. I felt chills run up and down my neck. "Daryl, I'll be back." I motioned for the women to follow me a second time to the central nursing station, out of earshot.

"He's awake!" For a moment, they stared at me in wonder.

"How can that be?" his girlfriend cried out. "We were told he was brain dead and that his heart and kidneys should be removed and given to someone...and that...and that..." She stopped, put her head in her hands, too confused to continue.

Yesterday, Daryl was assumed to be unresponsive. When coupled with the results of the scan and condition of the wound, his prognosis appeared hopeless to the attending physicians. More than 24 hours had elapsed since the injury; Daryl's brain had been exposed to the elements for an inordinate period of time. Infection was a distinct possibility. But all that was history now; I had to clean Daryl up and put him back together again.

"Since he is conscious," I told his mother, "we should give *him* the opportunity to decide whether or not he wants the surgery. Maybe he cannot tell us, but we should try to give him the choice."

"I cannot ask him. I just can't do it."

"Don't worry, I'll find out. First, I want to look at the wound."

I entered Daryl's room for the *third time*, and as the women waited in the far corner, I removed the absorbent towels from his head revealing several blood-soaked gauze pads. His shoulder-length hair was caked with brain matter. I put on sterile gloves and removed the pads. There was a circular defect in the bone approximately a half inch in diameter. I rewrapped his head with sterile pads followed by sterile gauze, placed my fingers in his hand, and bent down toward his ear. "Daryl," I whispered, "Squeeze my hand again."

He squeezed.

"Now let go."

He released.

"Lift your *first* finger," I ordered.

I removed my fingers from his hand. I watched a miracle unfold as he slowly raised his right index finger, just a tad, then let it return to the bed.

"Good. Now lift the first *two* fingers."

He lifted both in the same manner as before.

"Fine, Daryl, you're doing just fine. Now listen carefully. I want to ask you some questions and I want you to respond this way: if the answer is *yes*, then lift *one* finger. If the answer is *no*, I want you to lift *two* fingers. Do you understand?"

Without hesitation, his right index finger went up, then fell back.

"Do you remember me, Daryl? I'm Dr. Turner?"

One finger up.

"Do you realize that you are in Hilo Hospital?"

One finger up again.

"Do you know why?"

A two-finger response.

"Daryl, you shot yourself in the head. With a pistol. I'm sorry to be blunt, but time is critical. Because of the damage, you may never be able to move your left arm or leg again. Do you understand?"

He quickly signaled, *Yes*.

I repeated my question, "Do you understand?"

Again, he signaled with a *Yes* response.

"Ok then. What we need to know, Daryl, is...do you *want* to live? If so, I'll have to operate at once. So tell me, do you want to live?"

I didn't have to repeat the question again. Daryl lifted one finger for *yes*, then made a brief series of slow but definite finger moves: *one* finger, then *four* fingers, and then *three* fingers went up in that sequence. When his mother and girlfriend saw this, both of them burst into tears. I, on the other hand, was confused.

"What does *that* mean: 'one, four, three,'?" I asked.

"That's the beeper code the kids use: one, four, three, for 'I...love...you.'" The two women then hugged each other, their tears now tears of joy. Not only was Daryl still alive, he was not going to die. I excused myself to make a phone call. After scheduling the surgery as an emergency, I returned to cubicle 4B.

"Mrs. Ueno, I want to have a fresh flower arrangement placed at his bedside now, and throughout his hospitalization. I want to incorporate something called Johrei." I gave her an explanation of Mokichi Okada. She readily agreed. When I took Daryl into the operating room, the anesthesiologist, Dr. Steve Garon, moved several intravenous bags to their proper positions and helped me lift Daryl onto the table. He appeared irritated as he connected his machines and set the controls.

"Just what prognosis did you give the family?"

I put off answering my interrogator for a moment, knowing what lay behind his question. Only yesterday, Steve—while intubating Daryl—had been told that the boy was close to being brain dead. Later, when the mother declined permission for organ donation, he was asked to disconnect the respirator. However, after doing so, *he left the endotracheal tube in place*! That act alone saved Daryl's life. Perhaps Steve wanted to give him a last chance? Without the tube keeping his airway open, Daryl may have asphyxiated and died.

"Steve," I said, "It's a long story. Why don't I let Daryl answer your question?" I leaned down to his ear. "Daryl, open your eyes." He opened his eyes and looked at me. "Now look at Dr. Garon." He slowly directed his gaze to the face of an astounded anesthesiologist. "Do you have anything to say to him?"

Daryl responded with the *one, four, three* hand sign. Dr. Garon recognized the code and his face lit up.

"Steve, you saved his life when you left the endotracheal tube in his throat."

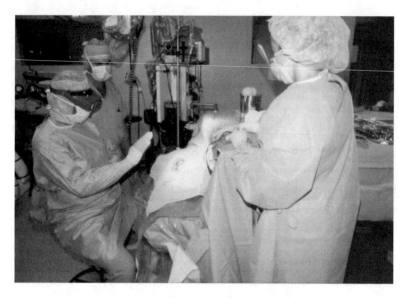

Giving intraoperative Johrei to Daryl

I began the surgery; the approach was identical with that of so many other craniotomies I had performed in the past. After removing the accessible bullet fragments, *debridement* (removal of devitalized tissue) of the wound and repairing the bone, I spent 30 minutes giving Daryl Johrei. Dr. Garon was seeing Johrei practiced for the first time. I explained to him that it was not *my* energy being transmitted to Daryl, but the *light* from Mokichi Okada, who currently resided in the spiritual world. He may or may not have comprehended; it didn't matter to me. I was more concerned with the outcome of surgery and Johrei than what others were thinking.

Daryl's recovery was astonishing! The day after surgery, his stepfather asked for a moment of my time. He had been in Chicago when Daryl was injured and when he heard what happened, he immediately returned to Hawaii.

"Doctor, may I ask you something?"

"Certainly," I replied.

"I was on the plane while you were in surgery. I just want to know if during the operation…was there a time when you thought you might have *lost him*? Was there a difficult time during the case?"

"Why, not at all. In fact, it went perfectly smooth. Why do you ask?"

"I'm afraid you wouldn't understand. Thank you for your time, doctor."

Within four days of Daryl's surgery—two days after I stopped the induced phenobarbital coma—an excited nurse approached me and reported that she heard Daryl singing in his room!

By the end of the second post-operative week, he was able to walk with assistance. His left arm remained weak, but he could manage lifting it to shoulder level. His speech was slow, but his words comprehensible. Each day, fresh flowers were placed in his room. He received Johrei twice daily from a MOA member. His supportive family always had someone at Daryl's side. In addition, they gave him nutritional supplements to augment the hospital food. When Daryl was transferred to a rehabilitation facility, he was able to sing a goodbye song of thanks to the ICU staff. Daryl's step-father again approached me. He was ready to confide why he had asked me that odd question about difficulties during the surgical procedure. When he learned about Johrei and another of my cases (which also involved light) in the ICU with Daryl, he knew that I would understand.

"You see, doctor," he said, "when I was flying back, over the middle of the Pacific, at about the same time you were in surgery, the cabin of the airliner suddenly filled with a brilliant white light. Nobody seemed to notice but me! Then, Dr. Turner, the light vanished as quickly as it had appeared. I thought this meant that there was a problem, that my son had died."

"As a matter of fact," I replied, "due to the time differences between California and Hawaii, I would estimate that at the time you saw the light, I was letting your son receive light from the spiritual world. *That blew his mind!*"

"Really?" he exclaimed, "you were doing Johrei then?"

"Indeed!"

He thanked me profusely and left with tears in his eyes.

Six months later, during a quiet evening at home, I was watching a movie when someone knocked on my door. To my surprise, it was Daryl.

"May I come in, Dr. Turner?" he asked.

"Certainly, Daryl," I replied, closely examining my unexpected guest. "His hair had grown back to shoulder length. He was well groomed and quite handsome. He watched the movie; I watched him. I was still amazed by his pseudo-resurrection.

"How did you get here?" I asked.

"I walked over; it's only three blocks. Thank you for saving my life."

"You're more than welcome Daryl. How is your left arm?"

"Oh, better, doc." He demonstrated by lifting his arm above shoulder level.

"Do you have any other problems?" I asked.

"Nope, none…except for the arm weakness and a little trouble walking. I want to invite you to a demonstration tonight. I have a new business, selling cleaning products, and," he looked around the room, "since you're a single guy now, I thought you might like to see some of our stuff. I'd be pleased to have you as one of my first customers. My friends want to meet you."

He handed me a business card and told me the time and date of the demonstration. I thanked him and assured him that I'd be there—not that I wanted any cleaning products. I was pleased to see him confident, happy, and back to work.

This was the story of young Daryl Ueno, a true miracle case. Exactly eight years after his surgery, Daryl came to thank me again. As we discussed the past, he remarked that the morning I saw him in intensive care, *he had seen me first*! He said that when I parked in the doctor's lot that morning, it was as if he were out of his body at the window, watching me walk into the hospital. He remembered hoping that I would hear about him and come to his aid. More importantly, eight years before his injury, he first started thinking about organ donation; it was frightening. At age 18, he remembered taking an automobile trip with a friend. During the outing he posed the question, "What if we got into an accident, ended up in a coma or something, and they thought we were dead and took out our organs?" Throughout the next several years, he had recurrent thoughts of being near death and having his kidneys removed. Because of this, he *never* wanted to sign an organ donation card. Lucky thing he told his girlfriend; the premonitions were words to the wise.

Daryl's story became the talk of the hospital. I was asked to give another seminar to explain the healing powers of flowers, natural foods, and Johrei. I did. As a result, several doctors and nurses received their o-hikari amulets and began to incorporate the medical art of Japan into their practices. It had indeed been *sandome no shojiki* for Daryl.

Chapter 12

The Angel
in the Light

Although there are families,
Each member has an individual life.
Man cannot prevent the inevitability of death,
Humans know this instinctively.

When facing the end of mortality,
All man can do is mourn death,
And take a moment to shed a tear.

Perhaps that is the reason,
I am compelled to do this.
Before displaying our grief over the passing of life,
We attempt to defy death's embrace.

At the very least,
We shall leave proof of the efforts made
To keep the dying ones alive.

And in these attempts,
As futile as they might be,
There is a glimmer of joy from the person
I have helped to exist in the world.

—*Blackjack: Clinical Chart 2* (Japanese anime video)

The first week after Daryl Ueno's surgery had been a period of illumination—a feeling of being surrounded by light. Not long after I had given light (in the form of Johrei) to Daryl, I was presented with a lesson about an angelic apparition appearing in the light. When something like this happens, is it a benevolent sign or is it ominous?

I met the Alvarez family the evening after Daryl's surgery. I was home, playing Chopin's *Ballade in G minor*, when the phone rang. Charles Benson, the ER doctor, said, "Jack, I know you are not on call…but I need a favor."

Someone is dying, no doubt. "Sure Dr. Benson, what is it?"

"The squad is bringing in a patient who had a seizure and now has a dilated right pupil; I think she has a bleed. Can you see her?"

"Of course. What time do you expect her to arrive?"

"In about 40 minutes."

Here we go again. "I'll be there shortly," I said. "Please notify the operating room nurse and tell her that I have a craniotomy to do." I intuitively knew that I would be required to operate on the unseen patient. I wanted no delays in getting a crew to the hospital.

Before getting into my truck, I looked up at the heavens. As if on cue, a shooting star appeared and made its brief transit across the zenith. I was growing comfortable with such signs, the advance notices of interesting things to come. I took this one to mean, *something amazing waits for you.*

At the hospital, Dr. Benson introduced me to Martha Alvarez, the patient's daughter, and handed me the scan. "This is the CT," he said. "It looks like a right-sided subdural."

He was right—a *big* subdural hematoma!

Martha Alvarez told me, "My mother was fine until six this evening. After taking a shower, she came into the living room and told us that she was feeling dizzy. She said that she had a terrible headache—then she passed out! We called 911. An intravenous line was started and just as they were putting her into the ambulance, she had a seizure."

I directed Martha's attention to the scan. The prognosis was horrible; Jordan Kalapana revisited. But what was this? Something was very strange. Her X-rays showed evidence of previous surgery: on *both sides* of her skull were single burr holes.

"When did she have brain surgery and what was it for?" I asked.

"A few years ago, she had two surgeries. We don't know the details except that the surgery was supposed to prevent her from having a stroke—she had suffered a few small attacks but they said they were transient." I knew what she was talking about. TIAs (transient ischemic attacks) where the neurological signs last less than 24 hours, and serve as warning: a permanent stroke may follow. "They also said it had something to do with her being Japanese."

I thought for a moment: *Japanese, small strokes, burr holes...*I'll bet she had a procedure for moyamoya disease! This is a rare condition, usually in Japanese females, that narrows a major brain artery. In addition, an abnormal network of fragile vessels forms at the base of the brain—these small arteries can rupture. On an angiogram, these vessels resemble a white cloud (in Japanese, *moyamoya* means "puff of smoke"). All of this went through my mind as I examined the films.

"Moyamoya, was it?" I asked.

"Yes, that's what they said!"

According to her chart, she only took medication for hypertension; her blood pressure at the time of transfer was high at 220/110. I directed my attention to the patient. I knew what I would find. Her right pupil was fully dilated. When given a painful stimulus, she extended both arms and turned the backs of her hands inward toward her body. This is an ominous sign called decerebrate rigidity, which indicates severe and perhaps irreversible damage to the brainstem.

At that moment Martha's father, Darnell Alvarez, appeared. I introduced myself, then said, "Why don't we step out for a moment?" But first I told a nurse, "Type and cross for two units. Tell the OR to send for her as soon as you have the blood drawn. Give her 100 milligrams of Decadron and a loading dose of Dilantin."

I led the Alvarez family to a small conference room at the end of the hallway and told them, "Mrs. Alvarez has bled into her brain, a subdural hematoma. It will have to come out. I have to move fast, turn a large flap of bone, and remove the bleeding.

The odds are against her surviving the operation. It is a serious bleed. I would like to be more encouraging, but now I must remove the pressure quickly to give her a chance." Darnell nodded but said nothing, nor did he display any emotion. I reviewed the surgical procedure and its risks. I told them that with the time delay (they lived in the country) more than two hours of valuable time had been lost since the onset of her coma. "I'm going to suggest that for a few days following surgery, she be kept under deep sedation. She will need her body cooled and that too has some risks, but we must take them. After that, I can try letting her wake up. I'll be able to tell you more then." I recommended that Johrei be added to her treatment, but the family *firmly* declined, stating that they had certain religious beliefs preventing such therapy. They said that they would pray for her.

"As you wish," I replied, my hopes that they would accept Eastern medicine dashed. I had no choice but to acquiesce to their demands. "I have to get started now; are there any questions?"

I was not prepared for their response. Usually, at this point, a family will say something like, "Please do all you can, doctor," or perhaps, "God bless you, we will pray that God guides your hands." Instead, the daughter said, "What about the light?"

"What light?" I asked.

"I guess that in the middle of everything, I forgot to tell you. This morning she awoke to the most brilliant light that she had ever seen."

"Interesting." I stood up to leave. "Be sure to tell me more about it. I have to get going if there is a chance to save your mother. I'll ask the nurse to keep you updated."

With that, I left for the operating room. It was all very strange. Yesterday, Daryl's father said that he'd seen a light in the airplane, and now this.

The surgery went well. I had no problem removing the clot. However, her brain reactively swelled with pressure and her pupil remained dilated. The ICP (intracranial pressure) monitor was reading high, and there were grave abnormalities in the waveform. I kept her in a coma with medication, using hyperventilation to reduce the swelling. I did not use Johrei. Only standard Western medical techniques would be used. I spoke with the family in the waiting room.

"Mrs. Alvarez has suffered a severe and most likely lethal insult to her brain. I believe that either the anastamosis ruptured—she had had a graft from an artery in the scalp to one of the brain arteries, as I understand the situation. It is also possible that the vessels near the base of the skull ruptured. The result was a subdural hematoma. She has severe brain swelling. We'll use all the means at our disposal to try and reduce the pressure, but her condition may not be reversible. Up to 10 percent of moyamoya patients die due to brain hemorrhage."

"What are you talking about?" her husband exclaimed. "They told us that after the surgery she would be just fine; as good as new and no more strokes." He began to sob quietly.

"Darnell, later, I want to explain about her prior surgery and Moyamoya, so that you can understand what has happened. There is a chance that she'll pull through, but it is slim. Do you re-member the Johrei therapy that I mentioned?"

"Yes, doc, but we are not interested. We will continue our prayer vigil."

The family, which had now increased from two to seven, thanked me for my efforts.

I kept the patient in a deep coma for two days. Each day after rounds, I would see Darnell sitting on the couch in the waiting area, his chin on his chest. I would sit down beside him and give him an update. On the third day, I reluctantly reported the sad news that *both* of his wife's pupils had become fixed and dilated, and the waveform from the Doppler (intracranial ultrasound) showed an alternating pattern suggestive of brain death. An EEG was isoelectric (flatline). Along with other tests of brain func-tion, the conclusion I reached was that Mrs. Alvarez had experi-enced irreversible brain damage. I explained this to Darnell.

"With tests confirming brain death, it is my opinion that there is no chance for her to recover. I recommend we stop the respirator and let her go."

"I *cannot,*" Darnell said. "I just don't know what happened and I don't know what she would want me to do."

"I know that this situation may not have come up for discus-sion between you and your wife, but I can advise you, as a physi-cian, that her condition now is beyond critical. There is no chance for her to recover."

"I don't doubt *you,* doc," he said, "but the problem is that I just don't know what to do. Do you think I could call the doctor in Honolulu that operated on her, to see what he would recommend?"

"I already called him. He is out of town until next week. I spoke with his partner, and perhaps you should speak with him."

Darnell agreed. This second opinion confirmed that his wife was beyond all hope.

"I *still* don't know what to do," Darnell said. "Can we wait until Monday, when the other doctor returns from vacation?"

"The decision to terminate life support is up to you and your family. We can wait."

At this point, his daughter came into the waiting area and sat down next to her dad. "Hello Martha," I said. "Could tell me about the light?"

"Yes, I wanted you to know. That morning, she woke up with a blinding light filling the room. She said it was so bright—so dazzling—that she had to cover her eyes. When she was finally able to peek into the light…she saw an angel."

"And then what happened?"

"She said the light and the vision disappeared as suddenly as they had come. Now here's the thing—my mother did something unusual that day. She went to a few friends. They said she looked more beautiful than ever before. In fact, she called one of my sisters—one who has been on the outs with her for two years—and somehow made peace with her. That night, in the shower, she felt the dizziness and…well, you know the rest."

"It's amazing that she had a warning of what was about to happen."

"Yes," Martha replied. "She described the angel in detail: wings, halo, benevolent smile—"

"Yes, but still, doctor," Darnell interrupted, "because we never discussed such things as life support, I have no idea of what she'd want me to do. Her surgeon will have a clinic in Hilo Tuesday. His office recommended that I call him when he arrives. They said that perhaps he could come to see my wife. Only 72 more hours. Can't we wait?"

We waited. The patient's condition did not change. Darnell remained morose. How sad it was that this man could not come to grips about what to do.

On the evening of the sixth day, I sat down with him. "Today was the doctor's Hilo clinic; did he get by to examine your wife?"

"His clinic was cancelled because of emergency surgery. It was like volts through my heart. I guess fate prevented his coming. Only God knows what I should do."

That night, at home, my gaze fell up on a book that my wife had given me a year ago: *Embraced by the Light*, by Betty Eadie. I realized in a flash that *this* book was for Mr. Alvarez! My eyes had been drawn to that small paperback, which seemed to glow in the dim light of the room. It was one of my books on near-death experiences and suggested that the spirit continues after physical death. It was a good personal story. I suspected that Mr. Alvarez could learn something from the author's adventure into near death.

The next morning, I caught up with him and said, "Come to the parking lot with me Darnell, I have something for you."

"Okay, doc," he said, his voice barely a whisper.

Outside, I handed him the book. "I think this may help you. My wife gave it to me, but actually, it was for *you*."

"Are you sure you want to give this to me?"

"Yes, I'm sure. I was just a go-between. It's *your* book." As I drove away, I saw him in the rearview mirror, standing in the middle of the parking lot, reading the book. Cars entering the lot swerved to avoid him. *Wow! He was into it.*

The next morning, as I prepared to leave home, I saw a ballpoint pen that belonged to my wife, a gold pen with a small angel on the clip (she was fascinated with angels). For some reason—one that would soon become clear—I put the pen in my shirt pocket.

As expected, when I arrived at the hospital Darnell was sitting on the same couch. He said, "Good morning doctor," and then resumed his usual position of despair. I sat beside him.

"You know doctor, all I could think yesterday was, 'Why is this guy giving me a book that his wife gave to him?' As you drove off, I looked at the cover of the book—*and I was shocked!* This was the *same book* that my wife had been trying to get me to read for two years, but I could not get up the interest. When I went home, I looked all over for that book, but I couldn't find it. Now I know—somehow, she used *you* to deliver this book to *me* so I would understand. *She wants us to let her go...to let her move on.*"

Without hesitation, I produced the pen from my shirt pocket and held it up so that he could see the angel.

"*Exactly!*" I said.

With that, Darnell's face brightened into a smile. He stood and extended his hand toward me. "Today, doctor," he said, squeezing my hand firmly, "this afternoon, we can discontinue the respirator. If you don't mind, there are two more family members flying in to say good-bye. After that, we'll be ready."

Darnell became a different person. He had a look of peace and serenity about him—an aura of contentment. He continued to smile. That small book answered his prayers.

Later that day, he called to say that the family had gathered in the room and they were ready for me to stop the respirator. I arrived moments later. In the room with him were his daughters. They had placed a tape recorder on a table by the bed. Darnell sat at his wife's side and held her hand, his head resting on the bedrail. The sisters nodded at me and then started the tape. I stopped the ventilator.

The song was one that I didn't recognize, but it was appropriate for what was about to take place. A woman sang to her lover of how he was her strength when she was weak; her voice when she couldn't speak; her eyes when she couldn't see; and how she would be forever thankful...because he loved her. It was Celine Dion's, *Because You Loved Me*. I was, like those present, moved to tears by the music and the sight of Darnell, holding his wife's hand...quietly weeping as the music played. I was not ashamed to have my tears openly displayed. To reach this point had not been easy for any of us.

Twenty minutes later, the cardiac monitor slowed to a flat-line tracing. It was over. Mrs. Alvarez had received a gift prior to her departure, a notice that gave her ample time to put her affairs in order—the angelic apparition. It was a good sign, that angel in the light. It gave her time to say good-bye, something that is not afforded to most people who suddenly lapse into irreversible coma and death.

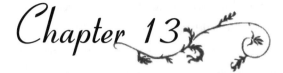

Chapter 13

Remote Viewing

Those who dream by day are cognizant of many things,
which escape those who dream only by night.

—Edgar Allan Poe

R emote Viewing (RV) is mysterious. It is a method of divination. At first blush, it seems like pure necromancy. But it is not; it is very real and it can be learned by anyone—if they know the method. As part of my investigation of unseen dimensions, the technique of remote viewing was a handy tool to have in my possession. I used it to visit the spiritual world, and for medical diagnosis. Remote viewing is simple to understand, effortless to learn, and easy to put into practice.

The three cases previously discussed (Mr. Sugitan, Daryl Ueno, and Mrs. Alvarez) suggested that the channeling of light from Okada, OBE, and contact between the living and the dead were not figments of my imagination; they actually happened. Now, as if these things alone were not strange enough to one trained in

Western science and medicine, more incredible and mystical events were to take place on my second trip to MOA zones in Japan.

I went as part of a group of doctors and ancillary medical personnel, all of whom had an interest in Johrei. There was nothing particularly remarkable until we reached *Kyushu* Island, where we visited a research center devoted to the scientific study of Johrei. Our group assembled in front of a Faraday cage—a room lined with layers of fine metal mesh—designed to prevent electromagnetic waves and electric fields from disrupting sensitive electronic recordings. Inside the cage, a subject sat with a full array of EEG electrodes attached to his scalp. The brain-wave tracings were displayed on a large projection screen. Dr. Rosenthal suggested we should direct Johrei toward the subject, hoping to see an effect on the EEG recording.

As the group extended their outstretched palms toward the observation window, I made a quiet and unnoticed exit to the adjoining conference room, where I waited for the next scheduled event. The bookshelves were full of texts on physics, medicine, and metaphysics. I took a seat at the table with my back to the bookcase. On a whim, I reached behind me and pulled out a book. I sat it in front of me on the table and with my eyes closed, I inserted a finger to a random page. I had selected *CIA-Initiated Remote Viewing At Stanford Research Institute.* I had at least 30 minutes before the others would arrive, so I dug into the article. This was my introduction to remote viewing.

In the 1970s, the U.S. Army became interested in Russia's psychic spies; the CIA became interested in mind control. The Army allocated millions of dollars to have Stanford Research Institute (SRI) figure out a method to keep up with Soviet parapsychology intelligence efforts. A famous psychic, Ingo

Swan, was part of the project. The resulting method was Remote Viewing, which produced results as good as any natural psychic could accomplish (with up to 85-percent accuracy). It was something that anyone could learn!

The *viewer* is given two sets of random four-digit numbers, which represent a "target." Starting with only these numbers, and by following a series of more than 200 precise steps, it is possible to download information from the "collective unconscious" (described by psychologist Carl Gustav Jung) that describes the target. The most amazing thing about remote viewing was that the designated target could be a person, place, or thing in the past, present, or future; all that is required is a brain and a notepad.

My friend, psychologist Dr. Don VonElsner, entered the room. "Don, this is something interesting." I slid the book across the table to him. As he began to read, physicians and nurses filled the room. While the Japanese scientists described their current research projects, Don's eyes remained glued to the book. He ignored the conference proceedings completely, never once looking up from the article. Dr. VonElsner—a brilliant and perspicacious man—must have found something of great interest. At the conclusion of the meeting, he approached me.

"Jack, do you realize…" He looked around the room and, after ascertaining that we were out of earshot, he uttered very softly: "I'll bet we can use this to play the market!"

I knew of Don's penchant for stocks and bonds and although I had no idea if remote viewing could be used in this regard, he was eager to find out. Although I didn't know it at the time, the great excitement that he developed over remote viewing may have been responsible for his demise.

Less than a week after my return from Japan, I watched a televised documentary called *The Real X Files,* the history of the recently declassified U.S. Army's remote viewing program. It featured Major Ed Dames, a former Operations and Training officer of The Defense Intelligence Agency's remote viewing unit. Dames recently formed a corporation with remote viewer Joni Dourif to privately teach remote viewing—for a fee. The following week, a friend phoned me.

"Hey, Jack," said the pleasant voice of O.B. Buckner. "Tell me something, what do you know about remote viewing?"

This was beyond amazing! It indicated that the next step was for me to become involved in remote viewing; RV seemed to be here, there, and everywhere!

"Well, it turns out that I *do* know something about it." I told Mr. Buckner what had happened that day in Japan.

"I have one favor to ask you," he said. "I want to drop off a tape and ask you to play it just before you go to sleep. Also, I need it back."

He must be talking about the documentary, I thought, but rather than admitting that I already had seen it, I said, "Sure, can you drop it off at my office?"

"Right on! You'll be astounded."

The package arrived within the hour. That evening, I opened the box expecting to see a videotape. Instead, I found an audiotape from an Art Bell (host of the late-night show, *Coast to Coast*) radio program—interviews with Emory University's Dr. Courtney Brown (a student of Major Ed Dames) on remote viewing. I started the recording and soon drifted off to sleep. I had a fretful night of strange dreams and awoke feeling that somehow, I had to learn the art of remote viewing. I remembered tiny fragments of the audio program—bizarre things about *pyramids on Mars; an Inventor's Hall of Fame; the Vince Foster assassination*—vaguely remembered fragments that were slowly fading away. However, I formed a conclusion based on what I had gleaned from the tapes: I decided that I wanted Major Ed Dames to be my teacher.

I scoured the Internet for information and read all that I could find on remote viewing. During my attempts to locate Major Dames, I learned that he and his company's vice president, Joni Dourif, loved Hawaii, but no contact information resulted from my search. Frustrated, I decided to train with Dr. Courtney Brown, lest the opportunity to learn remote viewing slip away. On his Internet chat site (The Farsight Institute) I met three people who later became my good friends: Martin Simmonds, Gail Harlow, and Dee Harris. Our chat group enjoyed discussing remote viewing and we anticipated exploring the world of RV together, learning how to put our minds in touch with the collective unconscious.

Then, one night, during a discussion on brain connections, Martin typed: "If a bird was sitting on the limb of a tree, and decided to fly away, would the bird fly up, down, or horizontally off the limb?"

I wondered why my friend has posited such a question, completely unrelated to our discussion. I took the bait, prepared for the yarn that was sure to follow. I made a stab at it. "The bird would fly up."

Before our eyes, we noted the sudden appearance of "FOX" on the screen with the response:

"Oh, that's known as alternative remote viewing, or ARV. It is a way of trying to play the stock market."

I flashed on Don's commentary about the market and remote viewing.

"Who are you?" I typed in.

"I work for Ed Dames at Psi Tech."

As we continued to text, I found that FOX was actually Joni Dourif, and by the end of the evening, I had a spot for private training in Hilo with Ed and Joni. I cancelled my scheduled training with Courtney Brown in Atlanta. This was exactly what I wanted, knowing that the apple never falls far from the tree. Ed Dames was the tree, and I wanted to be one of his apples.

Two months later, during the rainy winter of 1994, training with Joni and Ed began in my recording studio. The painting of the black lion with the red eyes overlooked the sessions, just as it did Gary Lyons's music years before. During the two weeks of intensive training, I encountered many weird and otherworldly events. My mind was sent from Easter Island to the boisterous and action-packed floor of the New York City Stock Exchange to the *Cydonia* region of Mars and to the *Santilli* Alien. It was a phenomenal experience. The training finished with my feeling comfortable with the ability to connect with the collective unconscious, where it is said that information is stored about every single thing known to humankind, in the past or present, and everything that will be known to humankind in the future. What an awesome ability to possess! But how could I apply it in my medical practice or in my search for the spiritual world? If RV could be used as an investigational tool for my interests, then I was ready to put it to use.

Chapter 14

The Scripter

The Moving Finger writes; and, having writ,
Moves on: nor all your Piety nor Wit
Shall lure it back to cancel half a line,
Nor all of your Tears wash out a Word of it.
—F. Scott Fitzgerald, *Rubaiyat of Omar Khayyam*

It came to pass that my RV Internet friends, Martin, Dee, and Gail arranged to meet me in Denver. During my visit, I enjoyed the kindness and generosity bestowed upon me by friends and family. This love provided fodder for a truly illuminating experience: the realization of how to accept and endure any hardship or mistreatment.

During the two years before this memorable trip in April 1997, I dealt with only one significant problem: relationships with women. I was working on my third attempt to have a meaningful and lasting marriage. I remembered the story of a man who always wanted to visit Hawaii, but was afraid to fly or to sail on a ship. He longed to live there, but his fears prevented him from going. One day, on a beach in California, he spied a bottle. When he picked it up and rubbed it, a genie appeared. In turn for releasing him, the genie agreed to grant the man one wish.

"Genie, I want to live in Hawaii but I'm afraid to fly. The engines can fail; there could be bombs on board. I cannot fly. And Genie, I don't like ships either. Ships sink. I want you to build a bridge from here to Honolulu. I want to *drive* to Hawaii!"

This stunned the genie. "Why, do you realize that the concrete...let me see, 6,000 cubic yards per stanchion and...not to mention 300 tons of steel for each 100 yards and...hey man, I'm afraid that's just about impossible, even for me! Wish for something else."

"Well," the man said, "there is one other thing that I want."

"Name it!"

"I've always wanted to understand how women think and how to get along with them."

The genie pondered for a moment, scratched his turban and said, "Before I start, I have only one question.

"What is it?"

"Do you want lights on that bridge?"

I too longed for an answer to those questions about women. I knew the answers were forthcoming, but it was taking a long time for them to arrive and waiting became a painful—and expensive—process.

I was having a rough go of it this third time around. On the occasion of a second period of rustication—trial separation—I had sufficient time to continue my study of metaphysics and spirituality at my country cottage. I read Okada's books on the eradication of disease, poverty, and conflict through Johrei. I read about his communications from the spirit world. Okada was certain that a plan for each of us is written in the spiritual world and that there is little we can do to alter it. Indeed, recent events seemed like I was merely an actor in a play. Tyrone's description of the Tree of Life had been helpful, as was my time spent with Buddhist chanting. Nevertheless, I remained at the mercy of forces obstensibly beyond my ability to control.

Two year previously, I discovered a brilliant essay by Mr. Okada entitled, *The Way for Man to Live* (from *Prayers and Gosanka*, Church of World Messianity, 1978), one of many *waka* (Japanese-language poetry) verses he created following his enlightenment. The final stanza was the key:

Let us have the strength
To bear with any hardship,
Any mistreatment,
Accepting it with a smile,
Just as though it were nothing.

Accepting any hardship, any mistreatment…that was it! I needed to be able to accept any form of mistreatment or adversity with a smile. Easy to say, but how could this be accomplished? Each morning upon awakening, I reflected on those five lines, hoping the answer to becoming impervious to stress would leap out and grab me. I needed to reach a point of peaceful coexistence with my wife.

Following the trip to Denver, I spent a few days in Ohio with family and friends. It was then that I suddenly became aware of—and fully accepted the meaning of—*The Way for Man to Live*. What if Okada was correct about life being a script that we must follow, and there is little, if anything, that we can do to change it? The struggles and strife we go through are lessons. If so, then what the hell had I been worrying about? The only choice (free will) that we have is how we will react to these events. Through a series of hardships (Okada called them "purifications"), we learn our lessons. Maybe we can only change how we *react* to situations. This was the hidden meaning in Tyrone's discourse on the Tree of Life when he said, "The choice is yours." Suddenly, I knew how to remain calm and restrained in the face of seemingly negative situations. It had required two years to raise my understanding to this level. It was an epiphany—and it came just in time, as that evening, when I called Hawaii to speak with my daughter, it was not my wife who answered, but my mother-in-law.

"Hello, may I please speak with—" She cut me short.

"That will not be necessary. You owe my daughter a divorce. I have ironed all of your clothes and moved them downstairs into the den where you may sleep on the hideaway chair. We want you out of the house. *We* want a divorce."

Had it not been for recent events, I would have lost my temper and given her a retort that she would not have liked. Instead, having reached that point of acceptance of events, I told her what she never expected to hear.

"Is that so? When I return next week, let's discuss it further, and see if we can reach an agreement about what I should do."

That was it! I *was* smiling. An important lesson awaited me, something that I needed to learn.

I returned to Hawaii three days later and took a taxi home from the airport. As we turned into the driveway, I saw my wife and her mother leering from the kitchen window.

My daughter ran across the driveway and jumped into my arms. "Welcome home daddy!"

Here was the only reason I came home.

I left two days later...never to return to cohabitation with my wife. I agreed to her request for divorce. It was with regret that I parted with my daughter, but I knew it would be temporary. What followed were several years of extreme stress in the form of legal entanglements. But thanks to Okada's advice— *keep spiritually clean and wait for the good things to happen*—I was able to endure the deluge.

I could accept that everything is written for us in the spiritual world, but something was missing: who was the *scripter*? I saw nothing to explain it in Okada's writings; I would have to look elsewhere.

At a neurosurgery conference in Boston, I fortuitously bumped into my friend, Dr. Melvin Whitfield. We took seats by each other in the meeting room. We'd been chief residents together during the final year of neurosurgery training, both of us African American. Melvin always kept his composure, especially at times when I reacted with irritation at events that seemed racial in nature. I am not proud to say that I was of this mindset. I have since learned to behave in a civil manner. One episode demonstrated how I reacted in my hot-tempered years and how, in contradistinction, Mel handled himself.

It was on a Wednesday, the scheduled weekly conference day, when the residents and staff from the departments of neurology and neurosurgery would meet. A medical or surgical case is presented to one of the junior residents and he or she would have to explain the case, discuss the radiographic findings, and recommend and defend a neurosurgical position on how to treat the patient. I arrived early, already upset, as I had watched the miniseries, *Roots*, the night before. I sat near two white women who were patients at the hospital and overheard their conversation.

"Do you remember the black man that took us to X-ray yesterday?" one woman asked.

"Yes I do!" the other replied. "He was tall and lanky, and I'll bet he can surely play basketball."

That ticked me off. To me, the basketball remark was a racial stereotype. The women continued to chat; I said nothing. When they left and doctors arrived for the meeting, I was in a foul mood. As fate would have it, I was selected to be the one put on the spot for the morning conference.

"Dr. Turner," said the staff neurosurgeon, Dr. Sadar, "let's have you discuss this case, a man with the sudden onset of severe headache and posterior neck pain."

I stood at the front of the room, 50 pairs of eyes on me, while a medical student put up a series of films on the view box.

I listened to the case history; it was obviously a subarachnoid (the thin web-like membrane covering the brain just beneath the dura) hemorrhage, perhaps because of rupture of an aneurysm or malformation of vessels. It seemed simple enough.

"All right," Dr. Sadar said as he pointed at the X-rays, "describe the blood vessels in the second radiograph from the left, top row."

I approached the view box and studied the vessels in question. "Those are anterior cerebral vessels. I announced, "and the—"

"Obviously," he interrupted, "but I'm referring to the tiny vessel, the one I think you'll find marked by an arrow."

"Hmmm," I replied, "I think that's the recurrent artery of Heubner, which supplies the head of the caudate and—"

"Nope, that's not correct." He smiled in anticipation of tripping me up further.

It was his remark, his tone, the miniseries *Roots*, and the ignorant women that suddenly made me confrontational. The keepers of my darker nature took over. I turned to Dr. Sadar and said, "I didn't come here to be played with. I am here to learn neurosurgery. I told you what I thought it was, and, if I'm wrong, then correct me. Teach me...but don't *fuck with me!*"

There was silence. Dr. Sadar and the others were shocked. A murmur spread through the room like a tsunami, then faded back into silence. Melvin, at the back of the room, covered his mouth with his hand and chuckled. That was his manner. Mel never overtly reacted to such situations—he always kept his composure.

Dr. Sadar cleared his throat, his face red with embarrassment. "Let's continue." He motioned to the med student, who described the surgical procedure offered to the patient. At the end of the conference, nothing further was said about the incident. Could this have been part of the reason that I was not offered a job in Cleveland after my training?

Years of being subject to racial prejudice had taken their toll. My fuse was short and it didn't take much to light it. I was sorry the explosion took place. Dr. Sadar was a likable guy.

Now, 20 years later, I found myself sitting next to Melvin at the conference, those training days long behind us.

"Hey, Mel," I whispered, "guess what? "I can now do what came to you so naturally. Whatever shit is dished out, I can accept it with a smile."

"That's right, Jack," he said. Then, with a knowing look he added, "Because you can't change it."

Melvin knew all along what I now realized after years of interlaced pain and suffering: it is written. Yet, I wanted to know exactly how is it written, and by whom? I would have to seek the answer from metaphysics, and in particular, from psychic research.

My search for the spiritual world had begun with an introduction to the spiritualist Edgar Cayce. Now, years later, I needed a more modern approach to the spiritual world so I could fit together the pieces of this enigmatic puzzle. Just as my interest in metaphysics began with Cayce's 1923 readings on reincarnation, my search would now focus on popular psychics who explain the spiritual world and the state of affairs after we leave our physical bodies. Their opinions are in keeping with the readings of Cayce, who felt that after physical death, the soul spends time on the spiritual plane, where decisions are made about further training in the form of "lessons" on Earth—lessons necessary for the soul's continuing education. Cayce believed that we choose when to return to a physical body, including choice of gender, and the re-embodiment would be among former friends and family members. The skills and special abilities that we develop during a lifetime on Earth are not lost, but carried forth into the new incarnation, albeit in a subliminal and subconscious manner.

Using the "retrospectroscope" (the answer to diagnostic dilemmas if viewed in hindsight), and looking back on the importance of Okada's poem, I realized that my reaching the point where I could bear any hardship and mistreatment (accepting it with a smile) may have saved me from serious illness or *dis*-ease. According to Gregg Braden in his book, *The Search for Zero Point*, an interesting paper appeared in *The Journal of Advancement in Medicine*, by G. Rein, M. Atkinson, and R. McCraty: "The Physiological and Psychological Effects of Compassion and Anger." They discovered that anger affected one component of the immune system (immunoglobulin S-IgA), and that for up to five hours after the inciting event, a reduction in S-IgA production could be detected. On the other hand, positive emotions led to a rise in S-IgA production that continued for six hours. The importance of this study is huge: self-induction techniques (to induce tranquility and peace) are useful in lessening the immunosuppressive effects of negative emotions. Had I not been at a point of acceptance that all is written, I would have erupted in anger when learning that, on my return to Hilo, I would be thrown out of my house. I may have (as portrayed in the movie of the same name), found myself *falling down*. My sudden awakening to the truth of how life operates prevented such a catastrophe. I felt blessed.

Much of what had happened up to now was based on faith—a belief in the opinions of others. I now faced the task of linking the common elements of the near-death experience, astral projection, and beliefs in reincarnation into a concrete and indisputable answer to the questions: Is there a spiritual world that awaits us after death? And in that world, do we ourselves fashion the plan for our next incarnation?

Comparing Edgar Cayce and Sylvan Muldoon to present-day psychics such as John Edward, Sylvia Browne, and Robert Bruce (who has published comprehensive books on astral physics) would provide enough information for me to form a conclusion. I turned to the psychics and to remote viewing for the answer.

Chapter 15

Out of the Shadows, Into the Light

Truth is simply whatever you can bring yourself to believe.
—Alice Childress

After vowing to incorporate Johrei into my surgical practice, I was made privy to many instances of patients whose illness, death, or recovery involved light. Okada healed with light; near-death-experiencers went into a tunnel of light; an angel appeared to Mrs. Alvarez in the light; and light flooded the airplane cabin, startling Daryl's father. What was the point of my light-related experiences? I pondered the question for some time and finally reached a conclusion: because our physical bodies are composed of light, it seems reasonable that our spiritual bodies will return to the light after death of the physical body. Hydrogen was produced as part of the Big Bang's primordial material; all the other atoms and elements in our bodies are from starlight—not from *our* sun, but a result of being forged in faraway stellar furnaces and reaching us by means of a star's terminal explosion. We are beings of light who have manifested in physical form. This return of the spirit to the light does not hold for the physical body. The atoms that comprise us will not be destroyed, but will go on (mindlessly) to do other things for all of eternity.

To verify my experiences to date as fact (my encounters with light and adventures suggestive of, but not proof positive for the existence of a spiritual plane), I turned to the metaphysical literature. In most religious beliefs, a higher power or benevolent force that is associated with light can be identified. Even the dark forces (for example, *Lucifer*, "light bringer") have been associated with radiance. Clearly, light was a connection to the spiritual world.

I now accepted as fact that all of our experiences, our actions, and perhaps even our thoughts are prewritten before our earthly incarnation. I discarded my attachments to karma and karmic retribution; those concepts no longer made sense. I wanted to know what was to come in the afterlife. I turned my attention to those who claim to have knowledge of the spiritual world, the people who profess ability to contact spirits of those who have gone before us: the psychics who claim to have knowledge of what lay beyond the darkness of the tunnel.

A chance Internet meeting with Australian psychic Robert Bruce was the catalyst for accelerating my investigations into the psychic realm. Robert is a skilled natural psychic who guided me to the study of consciousness and the seat of the soul. His book, *Astral Dynamics*, teaches the physics of the astral plane. Robert describes his "New Energy Ways" for achieving an OBE. Although I studied his work and was impressed with his detailed accounts of projection techniques, I had decided beforehand—after my lesson on the beach with Tyrone—to use enlightenment as a means to reach the spiritual world.

Sylvan Muldoon, Shirley McLane, Echo Bodine, Sylvia Browne, Robert Crookall, and scores of others describe the "tunnel of light" and the "other side." But what do we know about this dimension, both metaphysically and in terms of current physics? Bruce suggests that the tunnel is a *gateway* to other astral dimensions. The light at the end of the tunnel is the end stage of the transition from the earthly plane. A commonly held belief is that at death, the human spirit travels to a higher level through this tunnel.

All the psychics speak of what it means to go *into* the light. However, traversing the tunnel of light may not be a simple task. Mr. Bruce speaks of accelerating through the tunnel at a rapid pace and the ability to choose "exit points" based on perceived tones and colors. Can the soul have trouble reaching the light? I have one example based on personal experience demonstrating that at least one soul found this transition difficult. It came as the result of an extraordinary RV session.

During my remote viewing training weeks, I planned a wine and cheese party—many of my friends wanted to meet Major Ed Dames. Dr. Don VonElsner, the psychologist who was a skeptic when it came to spiritual matters, kept his hopes up that after I learned how to remote view, I would apply my skills to the stock market. He knew that I would be training under Dames and asked repeatedly if I could arrange an introduction. A week before the party, Don called me to ask how things were going. Ed and I were reviewing the day's training sessions when the phone rang.

"Hello, Jack, how's the training with Dames?" my sagacious friend asked. I could sense him straining at the bit to get on with predicting which stocks to buy based on remote viewing.

"Just fine, Don. I'm talking with Ed now." I told Ed that this was my good friend who was dying to meet him and would he take a moment to speak with him. Ed agreed. They talked for 10 minutes. Afterward, I asked Ed what he thought about Don's plan for playing the market. I was taken aback by his response.

"You were right, Jack, he *is* dying to meet me. And he *is* going to die."

"What?" *Bullshit!*

"He won't be able to handle the realization that remote viewing actually works. I had a similar case of a woman in Arizona, obsessed over the prospect of remote viewing. When she saw that it could be done—and that she could do it—she developed a high temperature that was nearly lethal. Her fever was unexplained by conventional medicine. Your friend is even more passionate about RV than she was. I am afraid he's going to die."

Utter bullshit!

I thought Ed was out of his mind. Although Don was elderly and had a bad back and other medical problems, he had no severe health problems. He went with me to Japan and kept up with the group of doctors without difficulty. He smoked, and also harbored an abdominal aneurysm, but he had been feeling fine at the ripe old age of 88. How could an intense interest in remote viewing lead to his death?

"Sorry, Ed," I said, "I can't agree with you."

Ed shrugged. "I have seen it before," he said.

Absolute bullshit!

The phone rang again—it was Don's wife. "Jack, something bizarre is happening to Don. Minutes after he hung up the phone, he lit a cigarette and began to tell me of his conversation with Major Dames. Then his hand began to shake and he turned as pale as a ghost. I'm worried. Can you take a look at him?"

Holy shit! Ed may be right!

"I'm on my way."

Major Dames declined to make the trip. Joni agreed to go with me. We arrived to find Don in his preferred easy chair, a weird smile on his face—a look of acquiescence.

"What happened?" I asked.

"Well, Jack," he replied calmly, "just after speaking with Ed, I sat down to tell my wife about our discussion, and I felt an extraordinary pain in my left arm."

"A radiating pain?" I questioned, thinking of a heart condition. "Any chest pain?"

"No, not that sort of pain, but a *strange* pain in my arm, much like the leg pain I had when I threw a blood clot years ago."

Don continued to display a twisted smile. I took his pulse, which was weak. As I palpated his heartbeat, his hand and arm slowly began to turn ashen and blanched as the blood flow decreased. He had thrown a clot to the *brachial* (arm) artery. I called his surgeon, Dr. Peterson. He told us to bring Don to the hospital; he would meet us there.

We wasted no time in getting Don to the emergency room, where Dr. Peterson admitted Don for evaluation and treatment.

It turned out that in the next few hours, the embolus cleared, the pain resolved, and Don was back to normal. This scared him. He vowed to quit smoking.

I returned home to tell Ed what had happened. His expression said, "I told you so." He could not be encouraging about my friend's future health. That extreme interest in remote viewing and the ability to see into the future, were what Ed considered to be the etiologic agents of Don's problem, not the smoking, as I had thought.

Don didn't make it through the next week. He developed severe abdominal and low back pain while out for a drive with his wife. He requested that she take him to the hospital. In the emergency room, he cried out in pain, a pain that required heavy doses of morphine. He made it through a CT scan that showed the aortic aneurysm leaking blood into his abdomen. Before any surgical intervention could be initiated, he died—in tremendous pain and discomfort. I received the call early in the morning and didn't know how to react. I was startled by the suddenness of his death. Though sad, I accepted his death as inevitable. He and I both knew that one day the enlarged vessel could rupture and take his life; still, I found it beyond belief to think it could be coupled with remote viewing.

In the days that followed Don's death, his wife asked me to present the eulogy at his funeral. I was in a saturine mood, but not excessively so. I recognized that Don's abrupt departure was part of a plan written for him in the spiritual world, and this plan could not have been changed. Still, Ed's words, "He is going to die," echoed unsettlingly in my mind.

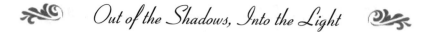

Ed agreed to go with me to the funeral. We continued our training as usual, and the last exercise of the day, about an hour before we were to leave, turned out to be of particular interest. Ed placed an opaque envelope on the table that contained a description of the target. He called out two four-digit numbers, and after copying them on the paper I began the mental process of downloading information from the collective unconscious. I drew and described a large structure—a cavern of some sort—cold, dark, and foreboding. In the cave was the target, a person seeking comfort and protection. Unlike other places that my mind had visited, this target site was a sinister one: a tubular structure with a faraway opening to the light of day. Yet this person—perhaps a shipwrecked astronaut—felt trapped in the cave. I saw no barrier keeping him inside. I sat back, dreamy eyed and still at the point of bilocation, when Ed spoke.

"I want to show you how to do a mind probe."

Following his instruction, I drew a schematic representation of this individual's brain and labeled the dynamic areas. I marked regions representing concern for family and friends; I labeled areas concerned with warmth, safety, and feelings of isolation. I pictured this fellow rubbing sticks, trying to start a fire. I felt the desperation and isolation that this individual was feeling. I paused, and prepared to stop. Then, something startling happened.

"What's wrong?" Ed asked, noting that my drawing came to a halt. I sat back in my chair and placed the pen atop the paper. A moment later, I once again took up the pen.

"I'm not sure. I wanted to stop here but something changed. I have the feeling that this person is asking me not to leave—*but to help*!"

"Do a mind query…another probe."

I began to circle an outsized area within the brain of the target, something active in the frontal lobe that was not present on my previous drawing. This area I labeled, for want of a better word, *telepathy*. It dwarfed the previous areas related to family, food, protection, and despair. "This man is now asking for my assistance, to help get out of the cave and into the light. He can see the light, but he's not able to reach it on his own."

Ed looked at me quizzically. "Stop and write your summary."

I wrote down the time and the word, *end*. On the next page, I wrote the summary:

> This person (a man) is stranded in a dark and cold place. He is dressed in white; he is unable to keep warm; he is concerned about his family and about sustenance; he can see the opening at the end of this damp and desolate cave; he feels utterly forlorn. He sensed my presence. He knew that I was about to end the session. He established telepathic contact, reaching out to me. In effect, he pleaded for my help and assistance. He wants out, but cannot find the means even though he can see the light. After he made telepathic contact, my feelings about this session changed. I no longer felt apprehensive or put off by the utter misery of the situation. I became willing to help.

"Is that all?" Ed asked.

"Yes, that's it. Perhaps an astronaut on Mars or something. I would never have thought that such an interaction between the

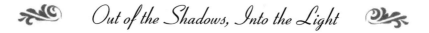

viewer and the target could take place. In neurology, there is something akin to this Ed; it is called *the feeling of a presence*."

"What do you mean?"

"People who have been left at sea in a lifeboat for days, often report that someone is with them, looking over their shoulder. A presence of another being is felt."

"Could it be some type of temporal lobe phenomena?"

I looked at my watch. I was almost time to leave for Don's funeral. "I would like to hash this over with you, Ed, but we have an appointment this evening. Later, we can talk about magnetic brain stimulation and Dr. Persinger's God-helmet experiments, but we're late. This was a strange RV session. Show me the target picture; I'll bet that you gave me a crash landing on Mars."

He did not answer. He handed the opaque envelope to me. I removed the folder, anxious to see the picture inside. It was empty!

"Where is the target?" I asked.

"You're right; it was a crash landing of sorts," remarked Ed.

On the tab of the folder were the two four-digit numbers: 7923 and 4852, followed by the words: *Don VonElsner: current status*. Never in a gazillion years would I have thought that Ed would have me run a session on my recently deceased friend, not in the face of the sadness that he thought I was feeling; and not just an hour before the funeral service! In retrospect, I now see how fitting Ed's request may in fact have been. Don, a "skeptic for life," was callously critical of any belief in a spiritual world. Ed knew that remote viewing was highly accurate—and perhaps precise enough to look into the whereabouts of someone recently deceased. It was an opportune moment for experimentation.

When I first met Dr. Don VonElsner I treated him for a pinched nerve and leg pain. He had mild post-operative tingling and pain that I thought would resolve quickly with Johrei. I told him about Mokichi Okada and the medical art of Japan. Though skeptical, he was willing to try Johrei. Ultimately he did a bit more than just trying it; he accompanied me to Japan, received the o-hikari and took part in channeling Johrei. I have him on video explaining that he was amazed to feel a sensation of heat emanating from his hand when he gave Johrei. He stressed the fact that the "psychologist" in him found it hard to believe.

Even though Don may have changed a bit after receiving his amulet, he remained unconvinced about the healing power of Johrei. He continued to scoff at Okada's writings on the invisible spiritual world. He often remarked that Okada was an accomplished "con man," as the MOA museums held many priceless pieces of art. Is it any wonder that after his death Don may have felt marooned in a place such as "The Holding Place," described by psychics like Sylvia Browne? Was he left high and dry in a queue of nonbelievers? It is within the realm of possibility to believe the self-proclaimed Doubting Thomas had been contacted by the process of remote viewing, and somehow communicated with me by means of an intradimensional conduit. A spiritual cord. As astounding as it may be, it appears that he had indeed communicated his urgent plea for assistance in reaching the light. My being there may have helped him. Now I would help him even more by delivering a stimulating talk to his friends.

The funeral went well. During my eulogy I was able to gaze at Don in the open casket, his o-hikari amulet around his neck. I saw Ed at the back of the room, listening to my words and knowing that his prediction had been 100-percent accurate!

I have described this remote viewing session to show that from this earthly plane, we can access those who have not made the transition through the tunnel and into the light. The Monroe Institute teaches how to assist such souls by using the Hemi-Sync *Gateway Voyage* and *Focus* audio programs that facilitate interaction with other energy systems (such as the afterlife). Would it be a stretch to believe it possible to remote view those who have passed into the light?

My interest and growing conviction in the existence of a spiritual realm sprang from what others say of this phenomenon, as well as from my personal experience drawn from remote viewing, lucid dreams, and miraculous signs that appeared in response to my requests. Having heard OBE accounts from patients who were never exposed to the literature and were unaware of the existence of near death experiences, I firmly believe that they were telling the truth.

In 2001, a PBS documentary described a patient of Dr. Robert Spetzler, renowned vascular neurological surgeon and director of Barrow Neurological Institute in Phoenix. His surgical team subjected patient Pam Reynolds to whole-body cooling, cardiac bypass, and EEG suppression for obliteration of a giant aneurysm of the brain (just as Dr. Hosobuchi had done for Rosemary). The patient recounted a typical NDE. I spoke briefly with Robert about this, asking him if he had previously been aware of reports of near death experiences and astral projection.

"Absolutely not, Jack," he replied. "I find it incredible that the brain can produce such events while in an isoelectric (flat-line EEG) condition."

Dr. Michael Sabom, author of _Light and Death_ and _Recollections of Death: A Medical Investigation,_ is featured on the documentary, displaying the craniotome that Ms. Reynolds described as looking like "an electric toothbrush." He shows the Midas Rex air-powered saw, which has a rotating blade, a slim cylindrical handle and could look like an electric toothbrush. Experts such as Madeline Lawrence counter that during anesthesia, the last of the senses to be disabled is the sense of hearing, and this could account for Pam's description of the instrument, a hallucination triggered by the voices of operating room personnel. But on questioning, the patient said that she never knew any neurosurgeons before Dr. Spetzler. Moreover, she was not aware of the design and purpose of the craniotome. As a surgeon, I acknowledge that we would not feel a need to explain or discuss the workings of the craniotome during a procedure. We would say to the scrub nurse, "Let's have the drill."

This case confirms the conjecture of those who say that consciousness may continue after the brain has ceased to function. Is consciousness distributed throughout the body's cells? And could this explain how Martha Alvarez directed my gaze to _Embraced by the Light_?

Remote viewing projects on life after death reveal that there is a spirit that lives on after death of the physical body. For example, a TRV training target given to beginning students was cued in a straightforward manner: "Human individual personality/ activity after physical death." I quote one viewer's analysis of her session. As usual, she was only given two four-digit numbers.

One thing I do know is this was a pleasant target to do, good feeling aesthetic impacts. There was a lightness about this target, a stillness that made me think of things such as winged angels and heavenly clouds. It was a target about a key to the way things are, or perhaps will be…why something works the way it does.

Remote viewing confirms what the psychics agree on, that the spirit survives after physical death. After a great deal of reflection on the pros and cons of the opinions of the psychics, the results of hypnotic regression, NDE, OBE, astral travel, and remote viewing, I formed my hypothesis: I am a believer in the life of the spirit that transcends our physical death, as there is more than enough evidence to support it. We are in contact with the universal force before birth, after birth, at death, and beyond death of the physical body. We can escape the wheel of reincarnation when we reach the level where we understand and can constantly practice *unconditional love*; when we have full realization that we are connected to the rivers that flow endlessly; when we see the miracle of the birds who fly through azure skies on bended wing, the trees that soar above us in majestic splendor, and all the earth's creations; when we realize that we share the same universal vital force.

Remote viewing was helpful in my investigation of the spiritual world. But would it help in the practice of medicine? Similar to how Ed used me to probe the afterlife, I would use Ed to probe an enigmatic case of unexplained post-operative pain. The session with Don is open to criticism, as there is no proof that Don was unable to reach the light. I wanted *verifiable proof* of the validity of remote viewing, something that I could see for myself.

Chapter 16

Medical Remote Viewing—
Medical Diagnosis

Remote viewing was interesting. It allowed me to tap the spiritual world and confirm its existence. But spirituality was only part of my interest; I wondered if RV could be of use in medical diagnosis. The period of training had presented a golden opportunity to find out. When Ed Dames and Joni Dourif came to Hilo to train my wife and me, I used my two weeks of vacation time to sit down daily and run training targets for several hours.

However, my mind was not completely devoted to RV training; there was a patient that I had operated on and discharged a couple of days before the training began. It was routine back surgery for a herniated disc and I felt the patient would do well. But I felt the need to keep in touch with him to be sure that his postop course was benign. I went to his home each morning, just to check. In the ensuing two weeks, the patient slowly developed a mysterious pain that was not revealed by his history or by my examination. I was stumped. Then, it occurred to me that I should run the cause of this patient's pain as a remote viewing target and see what Ed Dames could do to arrive at the answer. Not only would this be a confirmation of the power of remote viewing as a method of medical diagnosis, I would also have a chance to witness an expert at work. The results, as you will see, were everything I had hoped for; the patient fared well, much better than if I had tried to wait for the condition to become obvious on examination.

It was my turn to give Ed a blank manila folder. I labeled the tab, "Mr. W.D./cause of current pain problem." Ed took his seat opposite me at the table. I handed him a set of blank sheets of typing paper and a pen. Out of Ed's sight, I reviewed the patient's medical folder:

Mr. W.D. is a 58-year-old male who was first seen on April 10, 1996, for complaints of left leg pain, with left foot numbness and weakness. He failed to respond to conservative treatments of bed rest, physical therapy, and anti-inflammatory medication. A CT scan revealed a "soft tissue mass" to the left at the L4 level of the lumbar spine. A subsequent MRI

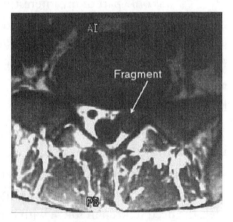

MRI showing disc fragment

clearly showed an extruded disc fragment at the fourth disc level (L4), with upward migration to the left.

The patient underwent microsurgery with complete removal of the disk fragments that compressed the nerve and were the cause of his leg pain.

Postoperative course:

Mr. W.D. improved and returned to his home state with mild persistent weakness of his left foot and mild residual numbness. He was re-injured months later when falling on his boat from his captain's chair.

Two weeks later, he suffered a twisting injury when working in the engine compartment. Repeat MRI scanning, with and without contrast agent, showed scarring and new extruded fragment at the fourth lumbar level. His left leg pain returned.

Microsurgery was performed and extruded disk fragments were removed. Considerable scar tissue was found as expected with fragments of disk embedded within the scar tissue. This required foraminotomy (removal of bone from around the nerve root). After surgery, his leg pain was completely relieved. He was discharged in improved condition. I will follow him with home visits or phone calls during the next two weeks as I will be out of the office.

Yes, that was the situation at the point at which I took a vacation to study RV. The patient complained of back pain during the first postoperative week. During my daily morning visits, he slowly developed shifting leg pain, the left leg greater than the right. But the next day, he would be pain free. Then, the pain returned. His temperature was normal and the incision remained intact—non-tender and normal in appearance. It was puzzling.

I arranged for him to attend physical therapy with heat, massage and ultrasound. Therapy helped him, but only a little bit. He felt that it offered "slight relief." I sent him to Dr. Greg Ruhland for nerve blocks, but steroid injections around the nerve did not change his pain.

By the midpoint of my RV training, the patient complained of pain in the front of his upper legs and in both calves. There was no evidence of venous clotting or inflammation. Straight leg raising (a sign of a pinched nerve) was negative. I was at a loss to explain his enigmatic pain complaints. It occurred to me that I could call on the universal force for assistance, not for physical aid, but for information. I would use this as a test case of medical remote viewing and run a session with Ed as the viewer. After all, why was I learning remote viewing if not to help others?

It is important to note that Ed Dames had no idea of this patient's history; he knew that each morning I visited a patient's home, but nothing of the man's history of his complaints.

I called out the numbers to Ed. He wrote them down and allowed his pen to make that first squiggle, an automatic response that contains all the information about the target. He went through the steps of decoding the tracing, steps that he knew well from his days as a training officer. He began to sketch and label the areas. He perceived the origin of pain within the brain and the source of pain in the lumbar (low back) region. That was interesting, as I had made no mention of the patient's surgery. As the session progressed, his sketches showed a tubular structure with a helical flow pattern and an obstruction to the flow by a reddish-brown material. Ed said that this substance appeared to be of fluid consistency.

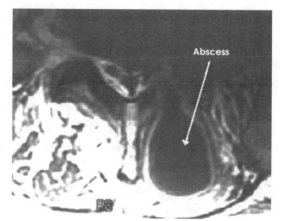

MRI showing abscess

According to the RV session, there was something obstructing spinal fluid flow in the lumbar spine. Was that something another extruded disk fragment? This was unlikely, as testing the patient by elevating his leg, a key sign of a compressed nerve, remained negative; if the RV session was accurate, it was not an extruded disc as the *nucleus pulposus* (the center of the disk and the part that ruptures) is the color and consistency of crab meat, not reddish brown. The bilateral anterior leg pain, when coupled with calf pain, was very strange. We concluded the session and I went to see Mr. W.D.

The patient had no fever. His back appeared normal. An interesting finding was his description of an area in the left lumbar region that, when pressed, would cause a radiation of pain to his left leg. I didn't know what to make of this. Based on the results of Ed's remote viewing session, I scheduled an MRI exam of his back. Something was causing nerve pressure and I could activate it by pushing on the muscles of his back.

On this scan, an isolated pocket of suppuration (pus) can be seen an inch below the skin surface and extending to the L5 nerve root. Needle aspiration yielded 4 cubic centimeters of reddish brown fluid. It was amazing! Ed Dames had correctly remote viewed the cause of the patient's pain.

I operated on the patient that morning, performing a surgical debridement under general anesthesia. A loculated area of reddish-brown pus was found, as expected. Cultures showed growth of coagulase-negative Staphylococcus (a common contaminant). I started the patient on intravenous antibiotics and twice daily wound packing and irrigation.

The patient made a good recovery, with the wound healing by second intention (filling in with granulation tissue and closing naturally).

This represents a case of postoperative infection that was a diagnostic dilemma for me, because of atypical symptoms and a fluctuating course of shifting pain in the back and both lower extremities. Examination of the patient's back gave no clues about the deep loculated infection. The incision looked entirely normal. The remote viewing session revealed anatomic features responsible for the patient's pain: obstruction of CSF flow by a mass lesion. This was a pocket of pus as defined by MRI scanning and needle aspiration. The diagnosis was reached by tapping the collective unconscious. This led to early treatment that prevented the infection progressing to the dreaded complication of severe osteomyelitis (bone infection) or worse. Had the patient remained untreated much longer, the abscess and low-grade bone infection might have progressed to a fulminating, and difficult to treat, osteomyelitis. This innovative modality—remote viewing—was an unusual addition to the holistic care of the patient.

Chapter 17

Now and Zen

A few minutes a day in total awe will contribute to your spiritual awakening faster than any metaphysics course.

—Dr. Wayne Dyer

With many experiences hinting at the existence of a spiritual world, a collective unconscious, and a universal force that can be called upon when needed, it was my goal to put the pieces together and form a conclusion about how things work. I reviewed interesting and relevant data:

Atheism can be defined as a disbelief in, or denial of, the existence of a God. Agnosticism is defined as being unknowing about God's existence or nonexistence. The following statistics from a recent poll taken by the *Wall Street Journal* explain what Americans think about God:

- 96 percent professed a belief in God.
- 90 percent said that they believed in heaven.

- 79 percent professed a belief in miracles.
- 76 percent reported a belief in the existence of a hell.
- 72 percent thought that angels are real.
- 65 percent felt that the devil is a real entity.

Education plays a huge role: 94 percent of adults without a college education believe in the existence of heaven; this percentage drops to 80 percent when college graduates are polled; it drops further to 75 percent when those who have obtained a Master's degree or higher are polled. It is interesting to note that 90 percent of American adults participating in a 1997 *Time* magazine poll said that they looked forward to meeting family and loved ones when they die. This group will be pleased with my conclusions. In a *Newsweek* poll that same year:

- 87 percent believed that God hears our prayers.
- 25 percent prayed at least one time per day.

Does knowledge of the cosmos or training in science influence theism? Also in 1997, a thousand scientists (members of the *National Academy of Sciences*) were polled randomly:

- 40 percent professed a belief in a personal God.
- 45 percent of mathematicians polled believed in God.
- 75 percent of physicists and astronomers did not believe in God.
- 69 percent of biologists did not believe in God.

- 79 percent of the physicists polled did not believe in God.

These illuminating figures reveal an interesting fact: *With increasing knowledge of science and astronomy, belief in God decreases significantly.*

Our knowledge of the universe has increased logarithmically since the mid 1900s, and an open mind—when cogitating on the conglomeration of astounding facts about the universe—will wonder what part he or she plays in the grand scheme of things. Our beliefs will be based on fact, rather than faith. Now, a decade or more after the previously mentioned polls, something interesting is seen. If education is *not* factored out, a *Newsweek* poll from March 2007 confirms that 91 percent of Americans continue to say that they believe in God, 82 percent identifying themselves as Christians.

In the beginning, there was the universal force. From this force sprang the cosmos, but in addition, many other universes—perhaps infinite in number—were also created at the time of the Big Bang. This initial energy may have been some form of "light," or perhaps nothing at all.

As our knowledge increases (and it is doing just that at an exponential rate), it will be interesting to see how our theistic beliefs change. Of all that we can see and detect, it is but 5 percent of the universe with 20 percent hidden from us as *dark matter* and 70 percent hidden as *dark energy*. When we learn more about this enigmatic 90 percent of the universe, many opinions may change.

Something of extraordinary significance occurred in early 1998: the discovery that the universe is not only expanding away from us, but has entered a phase of *acceleration* in its expansion. This implies that the universe may be infinite in extent, and the timing of this acceleration coincides with the emergence of human consciousness.

Just as I began to ponder the meaning of the universe, unexpected meetings with top-level physicists stimulated my study of cosmology (the history and structure of the universe) and cosmogony (theories of how the universe was formed). My oldest son, Matthew, alerted me one day by saying, "Hey Dad, you might like to know that Alan Guth will be on campus tonight." I was shocked! I had read Dr. Guth's book on the accelerating universe, but never in a million years did I think that I would meet him and pose a question.

Dr. Guth proposed the *Inflationary Model* theorizing that the universe expanded enormously within the first tiny fraction of a second after the Big Bang. Matthew and I attended his lecture at the Hilo branch of the University of Hawaii and listened with interest as he presented his theory to the assembled scientists. I had a chance to chat with him after his lecture. I wanted to know why the newly discovered *dark energy* was a repulsive gravitational force. He was able to give me some direction for study, but it was with the appearance of one of his fellow scientists that I came close to the answers I sought.

A few days after Dr. Guth's lecture, my friend Evonne asked me to stop by her bed and breakfast, *Hale Kai Björnen,* to see a little girl, the daughter of a mainland astrophysicist, who suffered from a splinter lodged in her toe. I left immediately for

Evonne's establishment on the ocean cliff, which was only two blocks away, and met the child and her father, who introduced himself as Michael Turner. He had been unsuccessful in extracting the foreign body and needed help. As we worked on the toe he looked as his watch, and I asked him if he needed to be somewhere else.

"As a matter of fact, I need to be at the hotel in 45 minutes."

"No problem," I replied, "I can handle this. By the way, what is going on at the hotel?"

It was then that I learned that Dr. Turner was a theoretical astrophysicist with Fermilab (the high-energy particle accelerator) in Michigan, as well as the chairperson of a conference on cosmology being held that week in Hilo. In one day I'd met two nationally renowned astrophysicists!

"What can I pay you for—?"

"There is no need for that," I interrupted. Then, as an afterthought, I added, "Come to think of it doctor, there *is* something you could do for me. I would love to attend this morning's session and hear your talk."

"Of course," he replied. "I'll leave your name at the door."

After removing the splinter from his daughter's toe, I left for the conference. Seated in a large ballroom I listened intently as Michael and others spoke of many interesting things, including the Hubble constant, the recently discovered dark energy, and the acceleration of the known universe. I felt like one of the "Three Princes of Serendip." How fortunate to be privy to this high-level talk and to sit among astrophysicists and astronomers of the highest caliber as they discussed my current interests.

Returning to thoughts on our composition (starlight), the elements carbon, hydrogen, oxygen, and nitrogen (CHON)—along with helium—were the early components of the universe. The remaining natural elements of the periodic table were forged deep within the centers of stars. The universe began from pure energy then evolved into mass, both the visible and the invisible (dark matter). That we are derivatives of this first energy, the universal force, may indicate that we connect with it when necessary. My final action would be to tie together the initial energy with what appears to be indisputable evidence that our spirit survives beyond death of the physical body. The question I put before myself was about consciousness and life's events. What state of mind is required to best get along in the world?

If we accept that life plays out according to a script written in the spiritual world, then it is not hard to achieve this awareness. It does not require faith; it is a matter of *waking up*. It is best to live in the *now*, being aware of every moment to the fullest. I quote Albert Einstein:

> The religion of the future will be a cosmic religion. It should transcend a personal God and avoid dogmas and theology. Covering both the natural and the spiritual, it should be based on a religious sense arising from the experience of all things, natural and spiritual, as a meaningful unity. If there is any religion that would cope with modern scientific needs, it would be Buddhism.

And this is correct: "Buddha" means "Awakened."

If you ask a number of people about their concept of Zen, you will get an equal number of diverse responses. There is a reason for this, but the reason cannot be understood unless you are living Zen. It is much like those who have experienced *satori* (sudden spiritual awakening). It is not something that can be put into words, but I will give it a try. In a sentence, Zen is an awakened consciousness, a change in the state of one's consciousness that allows you to be aware of what life is all about. In a word, *thus*.

I have included a few Zen references in the suggested reading section of this book. My initial idea was to explain why living Zen is the solution to a peaceful life, once one has accepted that all goes according to plan. I soon found that it is not easy to put such things down on paper. That is why Zen teachings are often in the form of *koans*—mysterious puzzles that have no answer. They are intended to spark awareness in the manner that a funny joke leads to sudden laughter. In like fashion, the parables of Jesus were designed to do the same thing: *wake us up*! However, in the case of the parables, the truth was revealed as well as hidden.

A koan example: There was a rich man who asked a Zen priest to prepare a writing, some type of scroll that he could treasure and could keep in his family forever; a memento of good fortune and wealth. The priest complied and presented him with a short parchment:

> *Grandfather dies,*
> *Father dies,*
> *Son dies.*

The wealthy man was outraged! "I asked you for something representing good fortune and prosperity and you give me this?"

"What on earth could be better than this?" replied the priest.

A parabolic example: *Isaiah 6:9–10*

⁹He said, "Go and tell this people:
'Be ever hearing, but never understanding;
be ever seeing, but never perceiving.'
¹⁰Make the heart of this people calloused;
make their ears dull
and close their eyes.
Otherwise they might see with their eyes,
hear with their ears,
understand with their hearts,
and turn and be healed."

I developed a great interest in Zen activities, such as the tea ceremony (*Chado*), Zen archery (*Kyudo*), and Zen sword fighting (*Iaido*), and the *Bushido* code of the samurai. I learned that the Zen mentality would keep the mind in great comfort, because this state of mind is the realization that all things are part of a divine energy: light.

From a scientific point of view, the concepts presented in two books on Zen and the brain, by James H. Austin, M.D., are points well taken. The effect on the brain of acupuncture, meditation, satori states, and more, are explained in great detail and worth studying. His work shows that there is *much* more to Zen practice than commonly thought by the average person.

It is said in Zen, that to put your foot on the path is the same as completing the path. It is easy to comprehend this meaning when one realizes the simple truth: the path is everyday life. And to best walk this path I was determined to find the missing link—the factor that I needed to complete my story. I needed to experience that connection with the universal energy, but not using an o-hikari amulet as in Johrei and the teachings of Mokichi Okada; and not through chanting, burning incense, and focusing on a Gohonzon, as in Nichiren theology; and not through the mechanizations and time-consuming techniques of remote viewing, but naturally—gathering and focusing the *Qi,* the vital force inherent in all things.

As if falling into place as the last puzzle piece, Qigong master Ken Cohen (previously mentioned by Mr. Kikuchi) was honeymooning in Hawaii and would hold a Qigong workshop near Hilo. I made plans to attend.

During that amazing weekend, I spent two full days learning primordial Qigong exercises as taught by an excellent teacher. According to Ken, Qigong practice leads to better health and vitality and a tranquil state of mind. Qigong practice allows us to control our reactions and reduce or eliminate disorders such as stress-related hypertension, frustration, and anxiety. I could feel this energy, appreciate its calming effects, and also its invigorating effects.

Qigong will be a powerful adjunct to my holistic treatment of the patient; it will act to enhance those skills that I have developed throughout the years. It was the missing link that I needed, not only for healing others...but also for healing myself.

Conclusion

Is there a single (creative) source of all that we will ever witness in our lives, in our world; is it possible that every life event, without exception, is part of that force?

—Gregg Braden, *Beyond Zero Point*

Alternative medicine, integrative medicine, and *complemen tary medicine* are terms that describe divergence from allopathic medicine. Hunter Campbell ("Patch") Adams provided care for the indigent and uninsured for years. He believed that laughter was the best medicine. As a neurosurgeon dealing with life, death, and potentially disabling and devastating diseases of the nervous system, I had little, if any, opportunity to pull out this *best* of medications from my medical bag of tools. Beginning with the standard techniques of Western medicine and science, I acquired additional instruments (alternative tools) to bring into the battle against disease.

According to R. Baker Bausell in his 2007 book, *Snake Oil Science,* it is not a question of *if* alternative treatments work, but *how* they work. Are alternative and complementary therapies effective due to the placebo effect? Is there another mechanism at work? These questions are important to investigators in the field.

To those of us on the front line who fight illness and disease, it is the outcome of our treatment that is of greatest importance, regardless of the method of operation.

"When you treat the disease, you win or you lose. But when you treat the patient...you always win!"

This statement, attributed to Dr. Adams, suggests that integrative medicine is best for the patient. Also, according to Albert Einstein, "Love is a better teacher than sense of duty."

I have presented many topics on spirituality, surgery, and integrative medicine, starting with events that led me to a path I follow yet today—the path to profound awareness of truth. I have described alternative methods of healing that blend with Western medicine. I chronicled my investigation of the spiritual world, consciousness, and the soul. The evidence for the spirit that lives on beyond death and beyond the physical body was presented as a series of patient encounters, some of them suggesting that a connection can be made on the astral plane, even in cases that meet the criteria for brain death.

The universal energy is present in every cubic millimeter of space; it is present in what was once thought to be the vacuum of the cosmos; it is present in the atmosphere we breathe. There is a never-ending drama of elementary particles that constantly spring into existence, which are then annihilated nearly instantaneously in bursts of energy. We need to understand that we are one with that energy and we are one with all things. What is *real* exists in the mind. The mind is *unreal* and exists in an indefinable and enigmatic dimension that we can only begin to comprehend. Our best course of action is to simply live in the moment and always do the right thing. When our time on Earth is finished, we are given the opportunity (in the comprehensive life review) to determine what is required on that long road to the point of perfect understanding. We have more polish to put on our spirit; we put together a new program of study; we return to complete our soul's education by the process of rebirth. After repeated incarnations, we reach the echelon of eternal spirits functioning in concert with the universal radiance.

But when on the Earth plane and our spirit has finally been forged from brass, tin, and iron, into silver and then to gold in the fires of trials and tribulations, and after we are given a shine, we must strive to, and direct all of our efforts to simply...*stay gold!*

Appendix

The Mind

I had been assuming that man is limited because his brain is limited, that only so much can be packed into the portmanteau. But the spaces of the mind are a new dimension. The body is a mere wall between two infinities. Space extends to infinity outwards; the mind stretches to infinity inwards.

—Colin Wilson, The Mind Parasites

An age-old question that at one time or another we have all asked—or it has been asked of us—is, "Have you lost your mind?" But, do we know where the mind is located within the brain?

The concept of the *mind* being generated within the brain is a topic that has generated much debate. The mind-body connection, the spirit (soul), and the concept of consciousness, are topics that were presented in the neurosurgical cases and personal experiences previously described. In order to understand the salient points of the previous chapters, it will behoove us to explore the matter of consciousness and the soul.

I have described patients who were in an apparent state of brain death (isoelectric EEG and lack of blood flow to the brain), and nevertheless recounted a NDE (as Pam Reynolds), or seemingly made contact with the physical world (cases of Kalapana and Alvarez). These stories raise interesting questions: do the mind and the soul live on past physical death? In life, where do we find the mind and the soul? What is consciousness and where does it reside?

The answers lie both on the surface of the brain (cortex) and deep within it.

Basic Brain Anatomy and the Theory of Consciousness

Much of what is known about consciousness is an enigma. It is difficult to investigate such a mystery when the analyst is an integral part of the mystery being investigated. The task of contemplating the mechanisms of the mind is a formidable one. The leading question that prefaces any discussion of the mind is where we *keep* what we so glibly refer to as a mind. Does it exist apart from the physical brain, or does it reside within the brain's substance?

Imagine if you will, a computer working quietly each night, trying to understand why it is able to compute. This is a formidable task for the computer, and it is an equally daunting assignment for humans to analyze brain function. Although researchers are making great strides in attempting to understand the mystery of consciousness, if there is a definite answer it remains tantalizingly out of reach. That is, out of reach if we try to understand the mind in terms of the commonly known three spatial dimensions. Clifford Pickover, in *Surfing Through Hyperspace*, quotes from P.D. Ouspensky's 1908 essay on the fourth dimension of space-time:

> We may have very good reason for saying that we are ourselves beings of four dimensions, and we are turned towards the third dimension with only one of our sides, i.e., with only a small part of our being. Only this part of us lives in three dimensions, and we are conscious only of this part as our body. The greater part of our being lives in the fourth dimension, but we are unconscious of this greater part of ourselves. Or it would be still more true to say that we live in a four-dimensional world, but are conscious of ourselves only in a three-dimensional world.

Our goal is to bridge the gap between brain and mind. If we can do this, we may have a chance to understand the mystery of life.

Consciousness appears to be dependent upon activation of widely separated areas of the human brain, rather than enjoying a special location within the brain, commonly referred to as the seat of the soul (or the seat of consciousness). It appears that the *thalamocortical* system and associated consciousness-specific interconnections with other consciousness-related brain areas might be responsible for conscious awareness.

1. Basic Brain Anatomy

The human brain, weighing approximately 3 pounds (roughly 2 percent of body weight), can be thought of as a sacrosanct vessel that contains and reproduces the world around us. All of our conscious and unconsciousness perceptions are filtered, altered, analyzed, and organized by a gargantuan symphony of neuronal elements. The resultant patterns are distributed to other body organs via nerve impulses and biochemical messengers. Our empirical universe is contained within the substance of the brain. There is a perplexing question generated by the study of the brain: What happens after the brain ceases to function and has surrendered to the dreaded ghost of impermanence? Is there something within the brain that lives on as the soul? Prior to a brief discourse on the origin of consciousness and the seat of the soul, it is appropriate to review basic brain anatomy.

The central nervous system (CNS) consists of the brain and spinal cord. This system is comprised of more than 100 billion neurons (nerve cells). In the developing embryo, a neural groove differentiates into a neural tube, and at the cephalic, or head end, the brain forms as the prosencephalon (forebrain). This is further subdivided into the diencephalon (midbrain) and the telencephalon (endbrain). When we think of the brain, we often picture two roughly equal-sized hemispheres, the inferior and posterior cerebellum, or "small brain," and the midline brain stem, which continues distally as the spinal cord. The forebrain is the most rostral (that is, closest to the nasal passages) portion of the three primary brain vesicles of the embryonic neural tube. The second major brain vesicle is the mesencephalon or midbrain. The third major division is the rombencephalon (hindbrain). The neocortex (commonly called "cortex") is a structure belonging to the forebrain. In the embryo of three-month gestation, approximately 250,000 neurons per minute are formed. At birth, almost the entire adult complement of neurons has been formed. At six years of age, the brain weight is one-half of the adult weight. At age 10, the brain weight is nearly the same as the adult brain and reaches its maximum weight at age 20. This increase in brain size is due to the rapid formation of new connections, myelination (formation of insulation) of the axonal fibers and growth of glial (supporting) cells.

The two grand systems of the CNS are the "motor" and "sensory systems." Muscular control (motor) requires many connections from the cortex of the brain to the basal ganglia, a term for the deep brain structures of gray (neuronal) matter, then to the cerebellum, and to motor neurons in the spinal cord and finally to the muscular system.

Incoming sensory signals (touch, vibration, pain, position sense, temperature, and so on), return via the spinal cord to the thalamus, the sensory relay station, and then to the cortex. Approximately 75 percent of the brain's neurons are located in the cerebral cortex, which contains billions of cells. The brain contains as many neurons as there are stars in the Milky Way galaxy and more than 100 trillion connections. The number of known particles in the universe is 10 to the 79th power. It is estimated that the number of *possible* neuronal circuits is 10 to the millionth power—a present-day computer cannot hope to compare. Current techniques of diffusion MRI with diffusion spectrum imaging (DSI) are producing maps of these interconnections as recently demonstrated by researchers at Indiana University; Ecole Polytechnique Fédérale de Lausanne, Switzerland; University of Lausanne, Switzerland; and Harvard Medical School. Their high-resolution map of the brain's cortex identifies a *network core* (located in the medial posterior cortex and connecting the brain hemispheres) that may lead to a partial understanding of the miraculous brain's circuitry.

The cerebral hemispheres are further subdivided into various lobes designated as: frontal, temporal, parietal, and occipital.

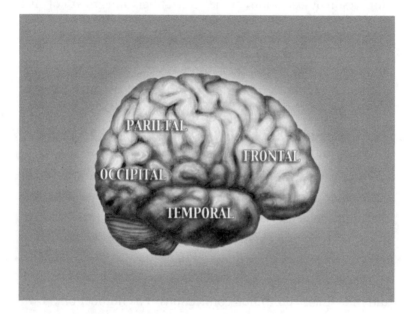

These divisions correspond to anatomical dividing lines based on various convolutions of the brain. Electrical stimulation of the pre-frontal area produces no motor movements and is called "inexcitable" cortex. The anterior frontal lobe is a location where intelligence was once thought to reside; however, with destruction of the area, there is no significant observable decrease in intellectual performance.

It is useful to think of the parietal lobes in terms of spatial orientation, speech, cognition, and integration of auditory, tactile, and visual memories. Various disorders of language, various apraxias (disorders of movement), visual field cuts, and patterns of body neglect are seen with damage to the parietal lobes.

The temporal lobe contains a preponderance of fibers involved with "facial recognition." Other functions include audition and balance, a portion of the pathways for vision and a portion of the olfactory apparatus for the sense of smell.

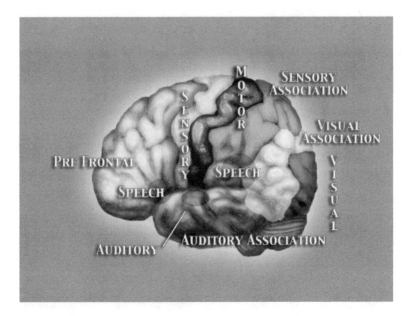

Key brain areas

Portions of the limbic system, which plays a major role in memory, are located within the temporal lobe. The figure shows key areas of the left hemisphere.

The occipital lobes are dedicated to vision and contain the pathways for visual perception and recognition. The next figure shows cortical landmarks, important fissures, sulci and gyri, and areas of the brain (cortical divisions) based upon known brain function. The frontal lobe lies anterior to the "fissure of *Rolando*" (central sulcus) and superior to the fissure of *Sylvius*. Notice how other fissures and sulci divide the brain into the parietal, temporal, and occipital lobes. The left hemisphere is shown due to the fact that speech centers are, for the majority of us, in the left brain.

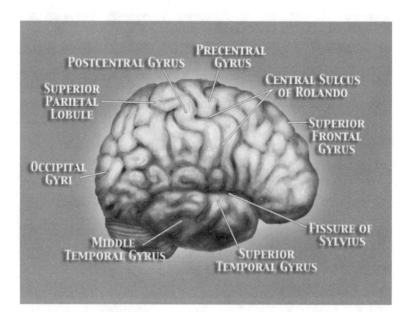

Cortical landmarks and brain function

The "motor strip" (motor cortex) is part of the frontal lobe, as is the "premotor cortex." The parietal lobe extends from the central sulcus to the occipital gyri. Below the Sylvian fissure is the temporal lobe. The cerebellum sits directly beneath the temporal and occipital lobes. In addition to lobar anatomy of the brain, Korbinian Brodmann (1868–1918) labeled 47 areas of importance (we now know there approximately 200) based upon cellular organization. Later, it was discovered that these are functionally distinct areas, such as areas 8 and 24 for contralateral eye and head movements, areas 44 and 45 of the dominant hemisphere (usually the left) as the centers for speech, and areas 17 and 18 of the occipital cortex for vision.

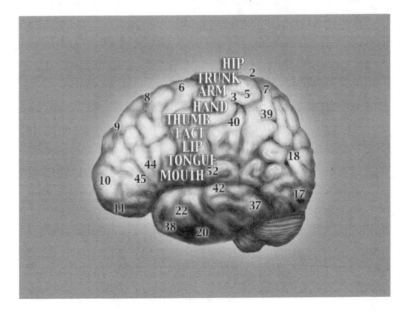

Brodmann areas

Brodmann's areas of the cerebral cortex were based on the cytoarchitecture (cellular organization) of each region. Within the cortical layers, *axons* (carrying the signal away from the neuron) and *dendrites* (fibers carrying incoming signals) extend vertically and horizontally, forming zillions of connections. There is a well-organized laminar pattern of axons and dendrites, with approximately 150,000 neurons beneath each square millimeter of cortex. The importance of this particular cortical architecture is the layering pattern, which gives the capacity to form the resultant huge number of connections; it has been clearly demonstrated to be a singular feature of the brain.

The cardinal feature of cortical neurons is their role in "mapping of areas according to function."

The right cerebral hemisphere, although somewhat larger than its contralateral partner, is a mirror image of the left. A thin but sturdy layer of dural tissue, the cerebral *falx*, contiguous with the hemispheric dura, separates the two hemispheres. Modern science tells us that the right hemisphere is the creative brain, and the left hemisphere the calculating or logical brain. Generally, language centers are located within the left hemisphere and important visual and spatial functions are contained within the right hemisphere. This is an oversimplification of what is an enormously complex system, but it will suffice for our purposes. The cerebral hemispheres are interconnected by the corpus callosum, a thick bundle of more than 300 million fibers. Deep within the brain are paired gray-matter structures: the thalami (sensory clearing houses), and parts of the temporal-lobe limbic system: the hippocampi and the amygdali.

The Mind

Why is the surface of the brain, the cortex, so unique? Just as an ounce of gold can be hammered into a sheet thin enough to cover a tennis court, the numerous foldings and enfoldings (gyri and sulci) of the brain allow a large surface area of the cortex to be compacted to the allowable space within the cranium (skull cavity). This outer cortical layer is very thin, varying from 1 to 4 millimeters in thickness, and is composed of more than 30 billion neurons, whereas the remainder of the brain and cerebellum has more than 150 billion neurons.

Within the white matter are the supporting cells of the central nervous system, the astrocytes, which nourish and maintain the neural cells and the oligodendrocytes, which produce the myelin sheaths of the neuronal axons.

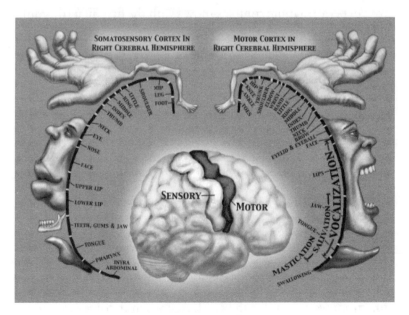

Homunculi

223

Astrocytes have been shown to interconnect with one another, forming even more potential connections that *may* be associated with consciousness.

The areas immediately anterior and posterior to the central sulcus are known as the precentral and postcentral gyri, and are responsible for sensory and motor functions respectively. The distribution of function is represented by sensory and motor homunculi (little men), and is drawn in a representative fashion; body parts may, at first glance, seem distorted and strange.

The relative size of each anatomical area corresponds to the amount of information being transmitted to or from the brain. For example, the area for the motor control of the thumb (right side of the figure) is far greater than that for the little finger, and we can perform more complex moves with the first digit (thumb), than we can with the fifth. The distribution pattern was obtained from brain stimulation sessions. On the left side of the figure, notice how the lips have a generous area of sensory cortical representation; that is indeed a fortunate evolutionary development.

Today, functional magnetic resonance imaging (fMRI), transcranial magnetic cortical stimulation (TMS), and other high-tech devices have replaced the direct brain stimulation for investigation of brain function. Edelman, in his book, *Bright Air, Brilliant Fire*, feels that there may be a large number of homunculi and that the visual system alone may have 30 such representations. Even though blood-flow studies and functional MRI studies are now shedding more light on the subject of cortical and brain function, we remain in the Dark Age when it comes to understanding the human brain.

11. Consciousness and the Seat of the Soul

The most merciful thing in the world, I think, is the inability of the human mind to correlate all its contents. We live on a placid island of ignorance in the midst of black seas of infinity, and it was not meant that we should voyage far.

—H.P. Lovecraft, *The Call of Cthulhu*

Aristotle (384 BCE to 322 BCE), thought the heart was the seat of all thought and consciousness, whereas Plato felt it was within the brain. In 1649, René Descartes, the brilliant French mathematician (he thought, therefore he was), described the pineal gland as the control center of the body and mind. Two schools of thought were established to explain the brain/mind connection. "Dualism" described a mind independent of the brain, whereas "monism" taught that the mind was located within the brain. Consciousness is the "active awareness" of one's mental and physical state, with the ability to transform these states.

Returning to the subject of the pineal gland, this structure is located at the apex of the brainstem (that is, the higher brainstem). Descartes wrote of *res cogitans* (thinking things) and *res extensa* (extended things) as components of the external world. The pineal gland was felt to be the organ that allowed res cogitans to interact with the res extensa. Although metaphysicians refer to the pineal gland as the "third eye" or "trap door of the brain," it is not tenable to think that the mind is located here. Melatonin and other chemicals are operational in the pineal, for light and time adaptation. As mentioned before, DMT (dimethyltryptamine) *if* produced in the pineal and released to bathe the superior and inferior collucli (connections for hearing and vision) during NDE and in death, may act to facilitate the transition into the light. DMT may be responsible for angelic apparitions who appear in the light and the mysterious light that can fill the cabin of an airliner. And, as Dr. Strassman speculates, the pineal may indeed be a trap door for entrance of the soul into the brain as it appears at seven weeks gestation (the same time that the sexual organs differentiate). Perhaps the soul enters on the 49th day and *this* is the true beginning of life. At death (or NDE), a release of DMT may occur to escort the soul back into the light.

There were many guesses as to the location of consciousness, but none seemed to be correct. According to Gerald M. Edelman, "Consciousness is neither a thing nor a simple property." Edelman has asserted that a fundamental property of consciousness is that it cannot be broken down into independent components. That is to say, consciousness is integrated within the brain, and involves many widely separated areas.

III. Electrical Brain Stimulation

On the surface of things, nothing appears as it is.
And yet, everything that appears unreal,
is more real than the surface of things appears to be.

—Source unknown

The work of Dr. Wilder Penfield, *The Mystery of the Mind*, will be instrumental in our search for the soul and the seat of consciousness. He realized that large areas of the cerebral cortex can be surgically removed without affecting consciousness, but destruction of small areas of the brainstem will seriously affect consciousness and can completely abolish it. As a practicing neurosurgeon, it was routine for me to care for patients who had sustained damage to the brainstem; consciousness could not be regained. In particular, when the reticular activating system in the brainstem is damaged, consciousness is not possible. Although traumatic unconsciousness may be caused by injury to this area, evidence points to the greater importance of diffuse lesions affecting the cerebral hemispheres.

The prefrontal and temporal areas at birth are two particularly important brain regions that are not initially dedicated to motor or sensory functions. Neurosurgeons are cognizant of the fact that surgical removal (or the old ice-pick *lobectomy*) of the anterior frontal lobe results in a decrease in the capacity for "planned initiative." Perhaps the elusive location of the mind is here.

Penfield noted that electrocortical stimulation of the brain yielded four basic types of responses: motor, sensory, interpretive perception, and recall of conscious experience. The temporal lobe was deemed responsible for "interpretation of present experience in light of past experience." Stimulation of the temporal cortex may result in the patient's experiencing dreamy states, due to the electrical activation of the sequential record of consciousness, as described by H. Jasper in *Epilepsy and the Functional Anatomy of the Human Brain*. These experiential responses were at first thought to come from a "memory cortex," but it was realized that cortical stimulation activated a distant secondary center of neurons in the higher brain stem (diencephalon). To explain this phenomenon another way, stimulation of the cortex does not activate neuronal cells in close proximity to the stimulating electrode (that is, the "local field"), as these neurons become paralyzed by the electrical current and, for a brief period of time, do not function. The signal travels to distant neurons in the spinal cord, termed "secondary ganglionic stations." (See Penfield and Perot's, "The Brain's Record of Auditory and Visual Experience: A Final Summary and Discussion," *Brain* 86: 595–696.) One of Penfield's patients described a "dreamy state," while her temporal lobe was being stimulated. She could clearly see and hear stored memories of her son playing outside the house, near the traffic on the street. Another patient unmistakably described his presence at a baseball game and his observation of a small child playing beneath the stands. Another patient distinctly heard an orchestra playing a melody. This was repeatable and unchanged with successive stimulation of the cortex. The following example illustrates some interesting experimental results:

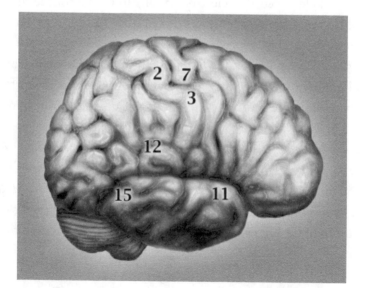

Stimulation point 2:	Tingling of patient's left thumb
Stimulation point 3:	Tingling of left side of thumb
Stimulation point 7:	Movement of tongue
Stimulation point 11:	Auditory memories of a conversation
Stimulation point 12:	Auditory memories of particular voices
Stimulation point 15:	Precognition of event

As a result of hundreds of brain stimulation cases, it can be concluded that the mind, and not the brain, "watches," and at the same time directs human cognition and function. If decisions regarding the target of conscious attention are made by the mind, then the mind directs the programming of all the mechanisms within the brain. Is there a "highest brain mechanism" that provides energy to the brain in a form that does not depend upon axonal potentials and flow?

Patients who were subjected to cortical stimulation that caused an experiential remembrance event were able to simultaneously experience the memory *and* discuss the experience. This is similar to the bilocation that is experienced during a remote viewing session. The viewer is keenly aware that he or she is sitting at a desk with pen and paper in hand, while at the same time being aware of a mental presence at the target site. Penfield labeled this experience of two streams of consciousness as "doubling of awareness." It was shown that the content of the dreamy state was dependent upon the concentration used, when the memory was recorded in the brain, and on which events were "paid attention to." Only events meeting these two criteria were "played back." He concluded that three integrative mechanisms were operational:

1. Highest brain-mechanism.
   —Located in the higher brain stem, a "grey matter" region (collection of neuronal elements).
   —Injury here can produce a loss of consciousness.
2. Automatic sensory-motor mechanism.
   —Coordinates previously programmed by the mind.
3. Experiential record.
   —Areas in the mid-brain and temporal lobe.

In two cases Penfield noticed that electrocortical stimulation produced a "forced thinking" intellectual aura. He concluded that electrical stimulation could not activate the mind.

The cerebral cortex is responsible for the "content" of consciousness. The reticular activating system is responsible for maintaining and activating a special system between the cortex and the thalamus. In this thalamocortical system, most of the neurons receive inputs from other neurons, not from the sensory system. A large part of the cortical activity is not appreciated as part of the conscious experience, although cortical activity is necessary in order for the conscious state to exist.

Strange things indeed occur. For example, approximately 150 milliseconds to 350 milliseconds prior to our conscious awareness that a voluntary motor act is about to begin, an evoked potential can be recorded from the scalp. Dr. Libet called this the "readiness" potential. Free and voluntary acts begin unconsciously, before awareness of the decision to act. Dr. Libet concluded that the cerebral initiation of a spontaneous act might begin unconsciously, prior to the awareness in consciousness that the act is already in progress. It begs the question, "Just who is doing the programming?" Libet does explain how there may be an element of free will that allows us to modify this process during a 200 millisecond period. However, if one is to make changes, the mind/brain must be ready to act in that meager one-fifth of a second. Mind-altering substances and lack of concentration may cause us to miss this window, the time when we can act to make changes. In *Scientific American,* August/September 2008, mention is made of a discover made by John-Dylan Haynes' team at the Bernstein Center for Computational Neuroscience in Berlin. Their work showed that in the prefrontal cortex, unconscious predictive activity occurs suggesting that indeed, unconscious brain activity occurs prior to conscious awareness and our actions stem from "preconscious brain activity patterns." This may not sit well with those who demand that there is such a thing as free will, but it appears that we may indeed be following a pre-written program.

Many years ago, my close friend Jim Brock called me to ask a question.

"Doctor, do you still drink?"

He knew me back when he was a Marine and I was a sailor. We were young and dumb in those days and we both drank like fish. But he had stopped using alcohol.

"Yes, mainly a bit of wine nowadays. Why do you ask?"

"Well, first, tell me doctor, why do you drink?"

"Well, it gives me a slight buzz; I don't drink to get drunk or anything like that, just a little buzz."

"Then tell me this, doctor, why would you want to change something—your brain and mind—that without drugs, is as perfect as it can be. The natural mind. Why would you want to alter it?"

I was nonplussed. He made a great point. The normal mind is a sharp as it gets. Everything else is a created illusion. That may be true when it comes to drugs, but meditation is something that can alter the mind in a beneficial way. In his book, *Tibetan Sound Healing,* Tenzin Wangyal Rinpoche explains it this way: "Ultimately, the practice (Tibetan sound healing) brings us to the full recognition of our true self. In the teachings, the metaphor for this experience is a child recognizing her mother in a crowd—an instant, deep recognition of connection, an experience of home. This is referred to as the natural mind, and that mind is pure. In the natural mind, all virtues are spontaneously perfected." Drugs may obscure the 200 millisecond window; meditation may help us to access it in time to make a change to what is already in progress; being fully alert and aware will let us take advantage of this small period of time and effect change.

One essential element for consciousness is the presence of "re-entrant interactions" for integration of various brain regions. This condition is felt to be a necessary, but not sufficient one, in order for conscious experience to take place. A study of the brain, during certain seizure states and in slow-wave sleep, reveals that the necessary conditions for consciousness may be satisfied, but the subject is not conscious. In sleep, the neuronal firing levels are similar to the levels seen during the awake and fully conscious state. It is the "pattern" of the neuronal firing that differs between the wake and sleep states.

- Waking state/REM sleep: The EEG shows fast, low-voltage waves indicative of many neuronal states. This is considered to be a state of "high complexity."

- Slow-wave sleep: The EEG shows a diffuse pattern of high-voltage slow waves. Global synchronization patterns are seen: A state of "low complexity." In this condition, consciousness is lost; brain areas are synchronized.

Consciousness requires continuously changing patterns of neural activity, and these patterns are spatially and temporally differentiated. This spatiotemporal integration of motor/sensory action is accomplished by "reentry" across brain maps. Edelman and Tononi postulate that the main mechanism accounting for neural integration is the existence of multiple parallel fibers with reciprocal connections between brain regions. We might ask: "What is the characteristic common to neuronal groups that acts to sustain the conscious experience?" Current research indicates that two critical items are necessary:

1. A dynamic core (neuronal) group, which constantly fluctuates in both integration and composition. It contributes to the consciousness experience through "re-entrant interactions" in the thalamocortical system, with a high degree if integration, reachable within hundreds of milliseconds.

2. This core, or functional cluster, must be of high complexity (that is, highly differentiated). This cluster cannot be broken down into independent components. Such a core changes in spatial location, composition, and time. This core cannot be restricted/localized to a particular position within

the brain. Such a system is termed "complex," which implies that a disturbance created in one part of the system spreads to involve (or to connect) all parts of the system. Consciousness is "integrated. "If the mind is the decision maker, then there is a back-and-forth interplay with the brain, which must act to store memories. Where is the energy source for the function of the mind? Can the mind be energized from power sources outside of the brain?

IV. Astral Dynamics and New Energy Ways

If the multidimensional nature of human consciousness is accepted, as can be experienced firsthand through the simple duality of the mind-split at close range, a great many complex issues and questions arise. These suggest the real possibility that multiple copies of the same mind can simultaneously exist on many dimensional levels.

Robert Bruce, in *Astral Dynamics*, asks, "What role do the astral planes play in researching human consciousness? Are scientists overlooking a valuable tool (OBE) that could complement EEG (electroencephalography), fMRI (functional MRI), and MEG (magnetoencephalography)?"

According to Rosemary Clark, *The Sacred Tradition in Ancient Egypt*, there is abundant evidence that the Egyptian belief was in the existence of multiple spiritual planes accessible from the material (physical) world, and the process of "transformation" was the technique to access these planes. The transformative processes were birth and death. Ms. Clark describes the *Ka* (Etheric Body), *Ba* (Astral Body), and the *Sa* (Life Force). The Sa was involved in all aspects of sentient life and was felt to be omnipresent in the physical plane; its function was to tie together the non-physical planes of manifestation. Understanding the relationship between OBE and physical body/brain memory storage appears to be the key to planned and repeatable OBE. Memory plays a crucial role, as the downloading of the projected double's "shadow memories" must take place to make these memories available to the conscious physical mind. If not, the OBE experience cannot be recalled.

The trance state is the first stage of a multileveled and multidimensional "conscious-exit" projection process. This allows waking (thinking) consciousness to continue within the confines of the etheric body, while at the same time, the physical body and its mind continue to sleep. The astral body, the next state of existence above the real-time body, maintains a center of consciousness that shifts from the real-time body into the astral body. The physical/etheric body conveys the majority of its energies to the astral body, thus allowing it to maintain full awake thinking consciousness. The physical body's original copy of consciousness stays firmly inside the physical body, but is energetically connected with its projected aspect at all times.

The Mind-Split: I had experienced that strange feeling of the *mind-split* during the bilocation of remote viewing. As I gained experience, a feeling of bilocation became not only familiar, but enjoyable as well (except for the initial apprehension I felt in the Don VonElsner session). What does modern science say about mind-splits? The *Ganzfield* stimulation experiment (that is, featureless fields of vision), where half-globe goggles of ping-pong balls are placed over the eyes and the face illuminated with monochromatic light, produces a sensitization to vision (similar to snow blindness) and consequently, perception is affected. For conscious visual perception, a variance in time must be present in the visual field. If a similar experiment is performed with goggles that project different stable and non-moving images to each eye, it can be shown that the mind cannot distinguish both images at the same time. That is, one of the images is selected by the brain to have priority, and that is the image that the mind concentrates upon, assuming the images are indeed incongruent. The *physical brain* cannot simultaneously be cognizant of both images. A form of complete perceiving can occur when the principles of the mind-split are taken into account and what in effect amounts to two pair of eyes are used. Muldoon believed this to be the case, and he termed the occurrence "dual perception."

Can consciousness continue to function in the physical body and the projected double at the same time? Muldoon and others assumed that the physical body was left behind as a "mindless shell" during projection. This was called the "empty-body assumption" and led to various beliefs that the physical body would require some sort of protection via amulets, incense, and prayers, during this "vulnerable" phase. Bruce assures us, however, that the physical body is quite safe, and a "master copy" of the mind remains securely within the confines of the physical body. Nevertheless, the physical body and the projected double must each be available for analysis of the "shadow memories" from the astral body, in order to perceive the mind-split that occurs during OBE.

The "energetic echo" is thought to be a reflected copy of consciousness, which can exist outside the physical body. This usually occurs during sleep and during an OBE, but may be a process that is unnoticed by the projector. That could explain my appearance in Rosemary's dream. The process can lead to the construction of *multiple reflected copies* of the physical mind, existing on different multidimensional levels. A master copy of the mind/memory/consciousness never leaves the living physical body.

The next immediate state beyond the physical body is the *expanded etheric body*, and works in this fashion: during sleep projection (or the trance state), a natural process occurs, as shown here:

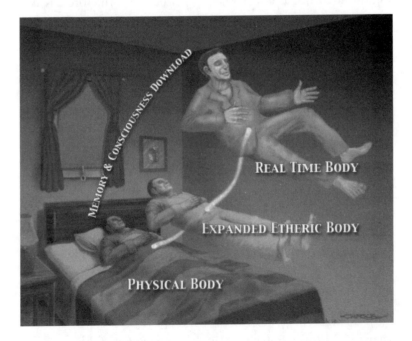

MEMORY & CONSCIOUSNESS DOWNLOAD

REAL TIME BODY

EXPANDED ETHERIC BODY

PHYSICAL BODY

The real-time body maintains a connection with the physical and etheric bodies, via the "silver cord." After projection, the real-time body is independent of the physical and etheric bodies.

It is capable of recording and storing memories, of experiencing and thinking. There exists a "sensory perception" interchange between the physical body and the projectable double, which decreases in intensity. Its maximum intensity occurs at a distance of 20 feet (according to Robert Bruce). It would be interesting to see if this varies with the inverse square of the distance between two points (d) as it should in a three-dimensional world. Or, does it vary as the inverse third power in a four-dimensional world? (that is, for a dimensional level (n), physical forces apparently correlate with the inverse power of the distance (d) according to the formula: $F = (K\Phi) / d^{(n-1)}$ where F is the force, K is a constant, Φ represents masses, charges, or other components, and d is the distance between two points of interest.)

The "mind-split" effect allows the animating spirit (soul) to exist in higher dimensions, being reflected from the physical/etheric bodies during sleep (Ouspensky's 1908 essay). From here, dimensions *beyond the fourth* can be reached through the process of *Multiple Mind Splits*, with each higher-dimensional body having a complete and fully functioning copy of the master (which is safely stored within the confines of the physical body).

Consciousness is a function not only of many areas of the cortex and the brain, but it also depends heavily upon the previously described thalamocortical system, as well as upon areas of the reticular system, the limbic system, and other key areas of the brain.

We have briefly touched upon "higher dimensions" in this chapter. Pickover states that, with the necessary folding of the human cortex in three dimensions, with its many gyri and sulci—which allow a tremendous surface area to be placed within the human skull—it is quite possible that our minds are likewise folded to the fourth or even higher dimensions. An understanding of OBE and the study of the astral planes may prove crucial to our understanding of consciousness and the human soul.

We have three methods by which to probe and investigate the astral planes:

1. Conscious and learned projection of the astral body (OBE).
2. As a natural consequence of enlightenment.
3. NDE.

Obviously, the method of using the near-death experience is not a viable option. The concept was explored in the movie, *Flatliners*. Method one, learning to consciously project, can be accomplished using a wide variety of teaching texts, from Carrington and Muldoon's seminal work, *The Projection of the Astral Body* to the New Energy Ways of Robert Bruce in *Astral Dynamics*. This leaves method 2, OBE as a consequence of enlightenment. This is the path I have chosen to follow.

My intent in the discourse presented in this conclusion was to describe the location of the mind within the brain and the probable mechanism of projection of the astral body, which could be a perfect tool to use to investigate the astral world. The investigations of Dr. Benjamin Libet in his book, *Mind Time*, show that the 350 ms period in which the brain is working to produce action, far ahead of our conscious awareness, is confirmatory evidence that we do appear to be following a predetermined script: one that was written in the spiritual world.

Further Study

Astral Projection

Bruce, Robert *http://astraldynamics.com/* (29 January, 2009)

The literature is extensive, from S.J. Muldoon, H. Carrington, *The projection of the Astral Body*. Rider 1929, to several contemporary books by Mr. Bruce including: *Astral Dynamics: Mastering Astral Projection: 90-day Guide to Out-of-Body Experience* (with Brian Mercer).

Astronomy and Astrophysics

Rees, M. *Our Cosmic Habitat*. Princeton, N.J.: Princeton University Press, 2001.

Coveney, P. and R. Highfield. *The Arrow of Time*. New York: Fawcett Columbine, 2000.

Consciousness

Dennett, D.C. *Consciousness Explained*. Boston: Little, Brown and Company, 1991.

Medicine, Miracles, and Manifestations

Further information concerning this book with discussions of stress reduction, life, death, and life after death, may be found at the author's Website: *www.JohnLTurner.com.*

Nichiren

A Dictionary of Buddhist Terms and Concepts by NSIC.

This is the best recent dictionary of Buddhist terms and concepts. It provides Chinese proper names, key terms, an Indic word list, Japanese equivalents, list of Sanskrit and Pali equivalents, and almost all the characters that are on the Gohonzon. It also provides the best and most objective account of other sects and practices.

The Threefold Lotus Sutra by the Rissho Kosei-kai.

Even though this is a flawed interpretation of the Lotus Sutra, it is still valuable for its "translations" of the "Sutra of Innumerable Meanings" and "The Sutra of Meditation on the Bodhisattva Universal Virtue."

The Liturgy of the Buddhism of Nichiren Daishonin by the Soka Gakkai.

This book provides the Chinese characters for the first half of the second chapter of the Lotus Sutra and the entirety of the 16th chapter of the Lotus Sutra. The Japanese version includes many Chinese characters of key terms in the silent prayer section.

Hurvitz, L. *Scripture of the Lotus Blossom of the Fine Dharma.* New York, N.Y.: Columbia University Press, 1976.

Prior to Watson's version this was the best translation of Kumarajiva's Lotus Sutra. Hurvitz includes a discussion of the differences between the Kumarajiva translation and Hern's translation from the Sanskrit.

Kern, H. *Saddharma-pundarika or the Lotus of the True Law*. North Andover, Mass.: Dover, 1963.

I love this translation from the Sanskrit. Its language is rich.

Soothill, W.E. and L. Hodous. *A Dictionary of Chinese Buddhist Terms*. Munshirm Manoharlal Pub Pvt Ltd., 2005.

This is a great book for understanding Buddhist idioms. An understanding of Chinese is essential to using this book.

Toda, J. *Lectures on the Sutra*. Tokyo: Seikyo Press, 1968.

A wonderful book by a person who lived the Lotus Sutra. It has a section of words and phrases of *Gongyo* as well as an interpretation of the silent prayers.

Watson, B. *The Lotus Sutra*. New York: Columbia University Press, 1993.

This is the most accurate and the most readable version of the Lotus Sutra in English.

Wieger, L. *Chinese Characters Their Origin, Etymology, History, Classification and Signification*. St. Paul, Minn.: Paragon Book Reprint Corp, 1965.

It is not as easy as a dictionary, this is a great source for understanding the radicals that compose Chinese characters. It has a few mistakes and virtually no understanding of Buddhist usage.

NSA on the Internet

Introduction. Imagery of Nichiren's Lotus Sutra. *www.gakkaionline.net/imagery/index.html* (20 April 2008).

Welcome to the new SGI-USA Website. Soka Gakkai International-USA. *www.sgi-usa.org/thesgiusa/index.html* (20 April 2008)

On the significance of the 108 beads on the prayer beads (Juzu): Billups, Alan. Juzu Beads and 108 desires. The New African and African/American Culture—Nichiren Soshu Buddhist Website. *www.proudblackbuddhist.org/juzu_beads_and_108_desires.htm* (20 April 2008).

Lotus Sutra

St. Clair, Richard. "The Wonderful Law of the Lotus Sutra." *Pure Land Buddhism. web.mit.edu/stclair/www/ lotus.html* (20 April 2008)

Neurological Science

Ramachandran, V.S. and S. Blakeslee. *Phantoms in the Brain.* New York, N.Y.: Quill, 1998.

Greenblat, S.H., ed. A *History of Neurosurgery: In Its Scientific and Professional Contests.* Park Ridge, Ill.: American Association of Neurological Surgeons, 1997.

Newberg, A., d'Aquili, E. *Why God Won't Go Away.* New York: Ballantine Books, 2001.

Philosophical

A Practical Guide to Death and Dying. Theosophical Publishing House, 1998.

Einstein, A. *Out of My Later Years.* New York, N.Y.: Philosophical Library, 1950.

Greene, B. *The Elegant Universe.* New York: W.W. Norton & Co., 1999.

Hawking, S. *A Brief History of Time: From the Big Bang to Black Holes.* New York, N.Y.: Bantam Books, 1990.

Hoagland, R.C. *The Monuments of Mars.* Berkeley, Calif.: North Atlantic Books, 1987.

White, J., Steiger, B. *Other Worlds, Other Universes: Playing the Reality Game.* New York, N.Y.: Doubleday, 1975.

White, J.W., ed. *Psychic Warfare.* Kent, UK: Aquarian Press, 1989. *The Meeting of Science and Spirit.* Paragon House, 1990.

Psychic Phenomena

Lerma, John. *Into The Light: Real Life Stories About Angelic Visits, Visions of the Afterlife, and Other Pre-Death Experiences.* Franklin Lakes, N.J.: Career Press, Inc., 2007.

Miller, Iona. Deep Field II: Entering the Earth (and DMT). *2007 Hyperspace Portal: PARAMEDIA http:// ionaparamedia.50megs.com/whats_new_10.html* (29 January 2008).

Ostrander, S., Schroeder, L. *Psychic Discoveries Behind the Iron Curtain.* Englewood Cliffs, N.J.: Prentice-Hall, Inc., 1970.

Rhine, L.W. *ESP in Life and Lab.* New York: The Macmillan Company, 1967.

Steiner, R. *At Home in the Universe.* Hudson, N.Y.: Anthroposophic Press, Inc., 2000.

Strassman, R. *DMT: The Spirit Molecule: A Doctor's Revolutionary Research into the Biology of Near-Death and Mystical Experiences.* South Paris, Maine: Park Street Press, 2000.

Qigong

Cohen, Ken. (Author of numerous books, audio CDs and DVDs on *Qigong*).

Remote Viewing

Sheldrake, R. *The Presence of the Past: Morphogenic Resonance & the Habits of Nature.* Rochester, Vt.: Park Street Press, 1988.

Wilhelm, R., trans. *The Secret of the Golden flower.* New York: Harcourt Brace, 1962.

Spiritual Healing and Alternative Medicine

Bausell, Barker R. *Snake Oil Science,* Oxford, New York: Oxford University Press, Inc., 2007.

Benor, D.J. *Spiritual Healing: Scientific Validation of a Healing Revolution.* Southfield, Miss.: Vision Publications, 2001.

Burr, H. S. *Blueprint for Immortality.* Trowbridge, Wiltshire: Redwood Burn Limited, 1972.

Guarneri, M. *The Heart Speaks: A Cardiologist Reveals The Secret Language Of Healing.* New York: Touchstone, 2006.

Matsen, J. *The Mysterious Cause of Illness.* Canfield, Ohio: Fischer Publishing Corporation, 1987.

Wanggyal, T. *Tibetan Sound healing: Seven Guided Practices for Clearing Obstacles, Accessing Positive Qualities, and Uncovering Your Inherent Wisdom.* Boulder, Colo.: Sounds True, Inc., 2006.

Zen Buddhism

Austin, J.H. *Zen and the Brain: Toward an Understanding of Meditation and Consciousness.* Cambridge, Mass.: The MIT Press, 1999.Suzuki, D.T. *Manual of Zen Buddhism.* New York, N.Y.: Grove Press, 1999.

Herrigel, E. *Zen in the Art of Archery.* Vintage Books, N.Y.: 1953.

King, W.L. *Zen & the Way of the Sword.* Oxford, NY: Oxford University Press, 1993.

Kushner, K. *One Arrow, One Life.* Boston: Tuttle Publishing, 2000.

Luk, C., trans. *Ch'an and Zen Teaching.* Berkley, Calif.: Shambala, 1970.

Suzuki, D.T. *An Introduction to Zen Buddhism.* New York: Grove Press, 1964.

Suzuki, S. *Zen Mind, Beginner's Mind.* New York: John Weatherhill, Inc., 1970.

Zen-Brain Reflections. Cambridge, Mass.: The MIT Press, 2006.

Index

About the Author

Dr. John L. Turner graduated from the Ohio State University with a degree in engineering physics, and continued in graduate school at the Ohio State University, Department of Physics.

Three years into the PhD program, he was given a book about Edgar Cayce, *The Sleeping Prophet;* this changed the course of his life. He was excited about the existence of a spiritual world and made immediate plans to attend the Ohio State University's College of Medicine where he earned his MD. He completed his internship year in general surgery and his first year neurosurgical residency at Ohio State University, Columbus, Ohio. He completed the remaining four years of neurosurgical training at The Cleveland Clinic Foundation, Cleveland, Ohio.

For 18 years, he served as the sole neurosurgeon on the island of Hawaii, initially performing lifesaving procedures with a marginally trained staff and substandard equipment. By all measures, Dr. John L. Turner is a surgeon with classic Western medical credentials. From his first day on call in Hilo, Hawaii, metaphysical events appeared for his edification and continue to the present day.

Throughout the past decade, the field of Complementary and Alternative Medicine (CAM) generated excitement as the next major source for improved better healthcare delivery. The aim of CAM (or *Integral Medicine)* is to use a complete and comprehensive approach in treating disease. This requires the practitioner to use many modes of inquiry to carry out the healing task. These modalities are grounded in empirical research and relate to models of human psychology, consciousness, subconsciousness, alternative medicine, Eastern healing therapies and the presence of a universal energy force. In *Medicine, Miracles, and Manifestations*, Dr. Turner utilizes this universal life force in a variety of nontraditional healing modalities.

During his career as a surgeon, Dr. Turner's curiosity drove him to explore several nontraditional healing modalities that broadened the scope of recovery for his patients. These new techniques included the practice of *Johrei* (the healing art of Japan), chanting and meditation (approaches found in all religious practices throughout history), soul travel and astral projection (as espoused by *Eckankar*, Robert Bruce and others), and precognition/remote viewing (as developed by Hal Puthoff, Ingo Swann and Russell Targ at the Stanford Research Institute).

Medicine, Miracles, and Manifestations, is the 20-year story of Dr. Turner's contributions to the field of neurosurgery through Integral Medicine. The concept of Integral Medicine has been written about by notable members of the medical community, including Andrew Weil, Larry Dossey, Deepak Chopra, Mehmet Oz, and Dean Ornish. Each of these writers is a physician who specializes in internal medicine. What makes Dr. John Turner similar to these writers is that he, too, is a physician. What makes him different from these writers is that he is a neurosurgeon. In fact, he is the only brain surgeon to write about medicine from this perspective: hands-on use of complementary techniques prior to, during, and after surgery, and exploration of pathways that lead to the spiritual world.

The tools of the surgeon normally have more immediate, measurable results on patients' health and well-being. With the opportunity to study and operate on the brain, Dr. Turner was in a perfect position to explore the mind-body connection.

Medicine, Miracles, and Manifestations reveals how metaphysical events such as remote viewing, telepathy, consciousness, and life-after-death are *verifiable manifestations* of the manner in which the human brain interfaces with the universal consciousness that author Lynne McTaggart refers to as "The Field."

Having reached the point in his life when could look back at his trials and tribulations, bless and release them, he realized the truth of the old adage, "When you get right down to it, if the mountain had been smooth, you couldn't have climbed it." As he encounters the interesting events and lessons that wait as he travels down the other side of the mountain, Dr. Turner enjoys a bucolic life in Hawaii. When not working as a medical consult or traveling to Japan, he spends his time with his wife Mikie and his small son Doushi, stargazing in his home observatory.